616.8'9   Novello, Joseph   996
Nov   The Short Course in
            Adolsecent Psychiatry -
            - Brunner/Mazel, c1979

DATE DUE	BORROWER'S NAME

616.8'9   Novello, Joseph   996
Nov   The Short Course in
            Adolsecent Psychiatry --
            Brunner/Mazel, c1979

THE SHORT COURSE IN ADOLESCENT PSYCHIATRY

The Short Course in Adolescent Psychiatry

Edited by

JOSEPH R. NOVELLO, M.D.

Assistant Director
Child and Adolescent Services
The Psychiatric Institute
Washington, D. C.

BRUNNER/MAZEL, *Publishers* • New York

Dedicated to my friends and colleagues on the staff of the Child and Adolescent Services of the Psychiatric Institute of Washington, D.C., whose dedication to our young patients and their families and whose unflagging pursuit of clinical excellence are a source of pride, stimulation, and continuing challenge.

Library of Congress Cataloging in Publication Data

Main entry under title:

The short course in adolescent psychiatry.

Includes bibliographies and index.
1. Adolescent psychiatry.   I. Novello, Joseph R.
RJ503.S48   616.8'9   79-681
ISBN 0-87630-196-0

Published by
BRUNNER/MAZEL, INC.
19 Union Square
New York, New York 10003

MANUFACTURED IN THE UNITED STATES OF AMERICA

Preface

This book is derived from a two-day symposium, sponsored by the Psychiatric Institute Foundation of Washington, D.C. While *The Short Course in Adolescent Psychiatry* is designed as a comprehensive review for psychiatrists, pediatricians, psychologists, social workers, psychiatric nurses, and others who customarily work with adolescents, we also hope that the book will serve as an introduction to the specialized field of adolescent psychiatry for residents, trainees, and others who have not known the joys of working with these exciting young patients.

ACKNOWLEDGMENTS

I am gratefully indebted to a number of people who have made this book possible:

Howard Hoffman, M.D., President of the Psychiatric Institute Foundation who encouraged the project from the beginning;

Al Bruce, Director of Public Affairs, whose sound advice and wry sense of humor only partially earn him the nickname, "Pesky Albert";

Miriam Mathura, Coordinator of The Short Course, whose organizational talents and steady reliability were just the tonic for the adolescent still lurking in me;

Mary Burnett and Brenda Loenichen who typed, proofed, retyped, cut, pasted, mailed, retyped, called, cajoled, and coaxed all of us along.

I would also like to acknowledge four very special people, former teachers and present colleagues, who have shaped and sustained my own interest in adolescents: Peter Martin, Derek Miller, John Meeks, and Reginald Lourie.

The contributing authors to this book are among the most distinguished experts in our chosen field. Their chapters will speak eloquently for them and for adolescent psychiatry. The opportunity of working personally with these men and women was my greatest source of pleasure in the project. We had fun—and we even met most of our deadlines.

My wife, Toni, has now been through two books with me. Always the pediatrician, she calls them "our surrogate children." She sees the whole process similar to a pregnancy: inpregnation; the first trimester when things are new, exciting, and developing rapidly; the second trimester of tedious boredom; and the final trimester when it starts to get painful and all you want to do is deliver it! Well, the labor and delivery are completed and we have the finished product, a surrogate child, in our hands now and it all seems worthwhile. Along with Toni and the distinguished contributors, I hope that our readers agree.

                                                    J.R.N.

Washington, D.C.

Contents

vii

Contributors

EVERETT DULIT, M.D., PH.D.
Director, Adolescent Psychiatry, New York Hospital, Westchester Division; Associate Clinical Professor of Psychiatry, Cornell Medical School, New York, New York

RACHEL GITTELMAN, PH.D.
Director of Psychological Services, New York State Psychiatric Institute; Associate Professor of Clinical Psychology, College of Physicians and Surgeons, Columbia University; Director of Psychology, Presbyterian Hospital, New York, New York

RICHARD L. JONES, M.D.
Instructor in Adolescent Medicine, Department of Pediatrics, Georgetown University School of Medicine, Washington, D.C.

EDWIN S. KESSLER, M.D.
Director, Children's Psychiatric Services and Clinical Professor of Psychiatry, Georgetown University Medical School, Washington, D.C.

WILLIAM M. LORDI, M.D.
Medical Director, Commonwealth Psychiatric Center, Richmond, Virginia

DONALD McKNEW, JR., M.D.
Staff Psychiatrist, National Institute of Mental Health; Associate Clinical Professor of Psychiatry, George Washington School of Medicine, Rockville, Maryland.

JOHN E. MEEKS, M.D.
Director, Child and Adolescent Services, The Psychiatric Institute of Washington; Associate Clinical Professor of Psychiatry, George Washington University Medical School, Washington, D.C.

JOSEPH R. NOVELLO, M.D.
Assistant Director, Child and Adolescent Services, The Psychiatric Institute of Washington; Assistant Clinical Professor of

Psychiatry and Pediatrics, Georgetown University School of Medicine, Washington, D.C.

DANIEL OFFER, M.D.
Chairman, Department of Psychiatry, Michael Reese Hospital and Medical Center; Professor of Psychiatry, University of Chicago, Chicago, Illinois

JUDITH L. RAPOPORT, M.D.
Staff Psychiatrist, National Institute of Mental Health; Associate Clinical Professor of Psychiatry and Pediatrics, Georgetown University School of Medicine; Subcommittee on Children and Adolescents for DSM III, American Psychiatric Association, Rockville, Maryland

REBECCA E. RIEGER, Ph.D.
Chief Psychologist, Chestnut Lodge, Rockville, Maryland; Former Chief Psychologist, Children's Hospital, National Medical Center, Washington, D.C.

ALLAN Z. SCHWARTZBERG, M.D.
Assistant Clinical Professor of Psychiatry, Georgetown University School of Medicine; Past President, Metropolitan Washington Chapter, American Society for Adolescent Psychiatry, Bethesda, Maryland

ROGER L. SHAPIRO, M.D.
Clinical Professor of Psychiatry, George Washington University Medical School; Faculty, Washington Psychoanalytic Institute and Washington School of Psychiatry, Washington, D.C.

ROBERT B. SHEARIN, M.D.
Director, Division of Adolescent Medicine and Assistant Clinical Professor of Pediatrics, Department of Pediatrics, Georgetown University School of Medicine, Washington, D.C.

PAUL S. WEISBERG, M.D.
Associate Clinical Professor of Psychiatry, George Washington University Medical School; President-Elect, American Society for Adolescent Psychiatry, Washington, D.C.

JERRY M. WIENER, M.D.
Professor and Chairman, Department of Psychiatry and Behavioral Sciences, George Washington University Medical School, Washington, D.C.

Introduction:
Adolescent Psychiatry Today

JERRY M. WIENER, M.D.

Disraeli, quoted as saying that "Youth is a blunder," captures the essence of one stereotypic view of adolescence—as a time of awkwardness, sensitivity, turmoil, behavioral and affective lability and unpredictability. As such it is best tolerated, lived through, and quickly forgotten in favor of later and supposedly better times.

Another familiar aphorism, expressing a related point of view, is that "Youth is wasted on the young." Here is a different but equally stereotypic view—adolescence as a special time of opportunity, vitality, exuberance, innocence and freedom, but, alas, unable to be truly enjoyed and appreciated by those who experience it. In this same vein, James Anthony (1969) identifies a number of other such polarized stereotypic views of adolescence held by adults, among them:

1) the victim vs. the victimizer;
2) as dangerous vs. endangered;
3) an object of envy vs. a hope for the future;
4) a bubbling caldron of sexual impulses requiring external constraint vs. a sexually inhibited innocent requiring external encouragement to be more "free."

Other views are presented in a variety of images offered on television, where the number of programs featuring the agonies and

xi

ecstacies of adolescence are meant to capture both younger children, for whom these images become role models, and adults, who readily establish identifications for vicarious gratifications. One need only think of the *Waltons, Happy Days, Welcome Back Kotter, James at 16* (whose first sexual experience became a national media event), and numerous others, to realize at least the breadth if not the depth of programming which reflects and exploits the endless fascination for adolescents characteristic of our times.

This fascination has been characteristic of psychiatry as well, including Freud's first case of a teenage girl with hysterical and conversion symptoms, and Kraepelin's description of dementia praecox, all the way to this Short Course in Adolescent Psychiatry, for which Dr. Novello has recruited a distinguished faculty to review our best current concepts of development, diagnosis, and treatment.

Of course, one presumes a more serious and productive purpose for this conference, for while everything always comes out okay for the adolescents we watch week after week on TV, in real life we know all does not come out okay. Indeed, we have reason to be concerned that, for a significant and increasing minority of adolescents, things are getting progressively worse.

A review of the reasons for this concern would include:

1) About 15% of our population are between the ages of 13 and 20, and it is a generally accepted estimate that 10% of these have some type of identifiable developmental and/or emotional difficulty requiring some type of professional or remedial intervention.

2) At a time when the number of psychiatric beds and hospitalized patients nationally is decreasing, the number of adolescent inpatients is increasing, and the percentage of beds they occupy is increasing.

3) Accidents, particularly auto accidents, are the leading cause of death in teenagers, with many left crippled when not killed. Considering the fearsome human and economic consequences to the individuals and to society, we have made relatively little progress in systematically understanding and/or using preventively those developmental, psychological, and psychiatric factors which surely play an important role in creating this carnage.

4) Related to the above, suicide is now considered the third or fourth leading cause of death in adolescents, and 20 to 100 times the number who succeed make an attempt or gesture, "cutting across" socioeconomic, ethnic, and diagnostic categories. What do we yet know about the antecedents, predictors, or prevention of suicide?

5) After over 20 years of experience in progressively refining the minimal brain dysfunction syndrome, or "Attention Deficit Disorder" as it will be labeled in *DSM III,* we are just beginning to learn something about its consequences during adolescence. As the myth that the symptoms go away at puberty is gradually dispelled, we have suggestions of outcome relationships to psychopathic and delinquent behavior, alcohol abuse, continued academic disability and depression. There is also evidence suggesting a genetic component in etiology and transmission in at least some cases.

6) Alcohol use and abuse and pregnancy in teenagers are increasing and are increasingly a source of concern. I mention them together because they both represent major public health problems with obvious ramifications beyond the period of adolescence itself. It was reported last year that in the District of Columbia the number of illegitimate births exceeded those in wedlock. When one understands that the majority of these illegitimate births are concentrated in the lower socioeconomic and disadvantaged population, one also understands the extent to which ever-younger adolescents' lives are prematurely careening off track. Further, there are increasing numbers of highly vulnerable at-risk infants who early-on become wards of society and later-on become disabled adolescents. So far the reaction of our government has been to discourage or prevent abortion, encourage sex education and hope that contraceptives will be used more often.

7) Serious crimes, especially crimes of violence, are increasingly a problem associated with adolescence. Sociologic and culture-related explanations are the currently voguish ways of understanding and explaining this phenomena, putting aside for the time being uncomfortable and, indeed, somewhat pessimistic insights and formulations obtained from the psychiatric studies of these adolescents. This studies demonstrate that serious ego deficits, character disorders, and developmental deviations are factors to be reckoned with in any consideration of prevention and habilitation.

Increasing numbers requiring psychiatric hospitalization, an increasing suicide rate, accidents as the leading cause of death, increasing alcohol use and abuse, an increasing incidence of pregnancy, more serious crimes and crimes of violence—this is only a partial list of the "slings and arrows." It is a rather gloomy and alarming litany, but one, I believe, which does compel and justify our concern and our professional attention.

At this point one is also justified in speculating about the relationship of these issues in adolescence to the changes that have occurred over the past 20 years in the ways we raise our children. For example, there is the increasing incidence of divorce so that anywhere from 35% to 50% of all children have experienced a broken family by the age of seven. Is it a cruel paradox that as we have become increasingly aware of the importance of early object constancy, attachment, and individuation for the development of psychological integrity and strength, other more powerful social, economic, and cultural considerations may be in conflict with the adequate provision of these early basic developmental needs? Is it possible that we are seeing an actual increase in the prevalence of narcissistic and borderline types of character organization, with their associated intolerance to frustration and conflict, impulsivity, need for more immediate and direct gratification, and impaired or limited capacity for sustained human relationships?

While it is one of the perogatives of an introduction to raise questions and leave the answers to those who will follow, I do not want to end on a note of pessimism. For there is also hope inherent in the driving, evolving dynamism of adolescence. In Sophocles' play *Philoctetes,* the Greeks banish the protagonist from their midst, and then discover that they must bring back this outcast if they are to triumph at Troy and survive as a society. The Greeks choose Achilles' adolescent son as their emissary; it is upon youth that they must depend for their future.

So it is also for us, as I introduce to you *The Short Course in Adolescent Psychiatry.*

REFERENCE

Anthony, J. (1969). The reactions of adults to adolescents and their behavior. In G. Caplan & S. Lebovici (Eds.), *Adolescence: Psychosocial Perspectives.* New York: Basic Books.

Part I

ADOLESCENT DEVELOPMENT

Part I offers the reader an overview of the "basic sciences" of adolescent psychiatry: developmental psychology, cognitive theory, physiology, and clinically relevant research.

Paul S. Weisberg, in the opening chapter, reviews the historical roots of adolescence and presents some provocative thoughts on why the nature and tasks of adolescence are changing. He also takes a clinician's view backward to observe that children *arrive* at adolescence today with new skills and vulnerabilities—and forward to observe that the life-possibilities in young adulthood and beyond have changed substantially. Dr. Weisberg summarizes the clinical implications of these changes and describes the new tasks that face those who would help adolescent youth.

In the second chapter, *The Three Stages of Adolescence,* Everett Dulit views adolescence from varying, but richly-integrated, perspectives: the descriptive perspective, the psychoanalytic perspective, and the cognitive perspective. In so doing, Dr. Dulit reviews the traditional stages or phases of adolescent development—with which all therapists working with adolescents must be thoroughly familiar. After reviewing the *science* of adolescent psychiatry, Dulit closes with a personalized view on the *art* inherent in the work of the adolescent therapist.

Chapter 3, *Puberty and Associated Medical Disorders of Adolescence,* is authored by two pediatricians: Robert B. Shearin and Richard L. Jones. No course in adolescent psychiatry could possibly be complete without a review of the basic physiology of puberty, but

1

Drs. Shearin and Jones go beyond these basics to also include an overview of common medical problems encountered by teenagers. Non-medical therapists are encouraged to be alert to the signs of physical illness in adolescents.

Daniel Offer in Chapter 4, *Normal Adolescent Development*, reviews some of his now-classic findings from his ongoing longitudinal study of normal adolescents and gives a glimpse at future directions. Offer points out that "only by understanding normal development can we understand its deviations."

1

The Changing Nature of Adolescence

PAUL S. WEISBERG, M.D.

In the past decades all of us have been witnesses to a historically unparalleled period of rapid change and loosening of security boundaries. The twentieth century has seen the end of empire and an extraordinary increase in the density of flow of value-threating and ambiguous information in each person's life. Consequences of these shifts, such as changes in social and political contracts and changes in the family's role, both to its members and in the larger community, have in many cases come to be accepted as normative.

We humans balance security interests against freedom-seeking interests in each of our choices. Many of these choices have become less socially defined, less obliged, and more individuated as the structure of social organization has loosened and the information flow has increased. The sanctity of marriage, for example, has traditionally operated in society as an organizing principle for behavior, a boundary against intrusion, and a security base. It has lost much of its power both because of a quantitative increase in the social tolerance given to alternate styles of adult living and because of the substitution of economic and security safeguards coming from the larger society for those formerly available only from the generationally persistent family. The breakdown of the consensual validations given to life long monogamous marriage has had a typical sequential pattern of a long period of eroding confidence, a relatively short period of revolutionary change in attitude (with the number of divorces

3

per year doubling from 1960 to 1972), and a final period of adaptation to that change. In this century, many other social and political systems, in analogous ways, have lost their power as behavioral organizers and security-givers.

To the adolescent, these change factors have had three prime effects: 1) The nature and tasks of the adolescent period of life have changed; 2) the skills and vulnerabilities with which children arrive at adolescence have changed; and 3) the potential outflow patterns *from* adolescence or, to say it another way, the possible integrations available to the adult as a product of adolescence have changed very substantially. It is difficult to define these very broad changes in anything like total scope. What follows will argue toward my understanding of how the psychiatric profession can impact on these issues; in order to define those impact routes, the problem areas will be outlined with what is necessarily a broad brush. I will, therefore, speak briefly to my understanding of these three major changes in adolescent life.

THE TRADITIONAL TASKS OF ADOLESCENCE

Before discussing the changing nature of adolescence itself in our contemporary world, it is useful and appropriate to review the traditional developmental tasks of adolescence. These tasks can be categorized thus: 1) There are tasks having to do with the adaptation of skills learned in preadolescent life in the small frame of the family and school to the larger conceptual and social environment open to the adolescent. 2) There are tasks which challenge the adolescent to adapt to a changed internal environment. Responses to newly-felt sexual impulses and increased motor capacities must be mastered, integrated, regularized and adapted to the adolescent's external life situation. 3) A third category of adolescent tasks has to do with attainment of a sense of personal autonomy so that the dependency need that is natural to childhood can be modified, adapted, or extinguished, and the person can become able to proceed into new life situations without undue fear of inadequacy. 4) There are tasks which adolescents face having to do with the achievement of intimacy with others, based on preadolescent affiliative skills and newly acquired autonomy, to the end that a reasonably consistent set of behavioral responses can be developed with another. This involves a partial and voluntary diminution of the boundary systems which in each of us separates the self from the non-self. 5) Finally, the adolescent faces a set of tasks which has to do with adaptation to the work function in society, with the establishment of persistent goals and a focus on acquisition of necessary work skills to achieve those goals. Some of these tasks overlap, both in time and in function, but the accomplishment of each of them, and the integration into the self of the resultant states of coping adequacy, are necessary for the adolescent to arrive successfully at competent adulthood.

One more categorical distinction in the nature of adolescent function will be mentioned, which is the fact that this is a developmental model. This developmental model combines with the task model outlined above to give the observer a stereoscopic perception of adolescent function. Developmentally, adolescence can be divided into three subperiods: early, middle and late.

Early Adolescence

The first subperiod, ordinarily lasting from about age 12 through about age 14, can be thought of as the period of immediate responses to puberty. During this period there is ordinarily a high level of residual dependency on the family or family surrogate, a high level of discomfort and changed bodily function, a high proclivity to feelings of shame inside the family, a proclivity to psychosomatic expressions of anxiety, and a reorganization of peer affiliations.

Middle Adolescence

In middle adolescence, lasting from about the fifteenth to the seventeenth birthdays, there is ordinarily a maximization of rebellion against parental values; a high degree of use of the peer group as a family substitute in value acquisition; a high degree of idealism based on vulnerability (which is, in fact, largely a projection of internally perceived inabilities to cope without family protection); substantial use of available, socially disapproved substances, such as drugs and alcohol, both to relieve anxiety and to achieve a magical sense of power; a tendency to test legal and moral boundaries with antisocial behavior such as stealing or promiscuity; and a utilization of alternate adult figures as identification models, these adults serving both as objective representatives of society and as parent surrogates.

Late Adolescence

Late adolescence, lasting ordinarily from about the seventeenth birthday until identity formation is reasonably complete, has as its cardinal features the partial giving up of negativistic behavior; an increasing sense of personality integration; a transmutation of goals from the rebellious, "hiding out" ones of middle adolescence to future-oriented ones; the establishment of transient but deepening heterosexual intimacy; and the acquisition and solidification of work skills.

These developmental distinctions are important in understanding the role of the family during adolescence, the nature of the need that the adolescent presents to a psychiatric examiner at any point during the adolescent process, and the deficits that an adolescent of any given age possesses in terms of incomplete accomplishment of previous tasks necessary to ready him or her for the age-appropriate tasks at hand.

THE CHANGING NATURE OF ADOLESCENCE ITSELF

Adolescence has been described as a period of life which begins with a physical event, that is, puberty, and ends with a psychological one, that is, the formation of an adult identity. Puberty's nature has changed little, if at all, in our time, although there has been, in developed nations, a consistent lowering of the median age of puberty over the past 100 years. The nature of adolescence, however, has changed in its focus. In an agrarian society adolescence was minimal and transient as a definable period. Industrial societies, however, because of the nature of their organization, required specialized work skills and highly integrated patterns of social adaptation to an urban and often a corporate setting to function efficiently. To that end, a system evolved through the nineteenth and early twentieth centuries, which was characterized by delay of assumption of adult responsibilities while the adolescent pursued the tasks of achieving a separation from family that was psychological without being physical. Barriers were created against adolescent heterosexual intimacy, while acquisition of sophisticated work skills was emphasized. This system, called "adolescence," introduced new stresses through its imposition, on a large scale, of delay in sexual and aggressive outlet and its enforcement of regressed child-appropriate standards of autonomy during a period of physical and conceptual maturity. It also led to enormous technical and economic progress, through the creation of a skilled and, at times, even educated populace. Adolescence, as a system, has entered the same eroding phase in this country as have so many of our other systems, with loss of consensual validation stemming from the lessening of the social needs that adolescence filled. It is an idea whose time has passed. A highly skilled populace has less social and economic importance as machines are developed that solve concrete problems and produce goods with greater speed and efficiency than can humans. Conceptualization of problems remains an important human task, but as computer hardware and programs are developed which make solutions to more and more complex problems increasingly available, the time grows closer when human conceptual decision-making will become less efficient than that of the computer in most areas. For much of this nation's population that is now adolescent, early retirement or another form of a lengthy non-work status during their lives is probable.

While the economic advantages of adolescence are in decline, the social ones of increased interpersonal skill development remain and, in many ways, have become more important. The breaking down of that part of the social system called adolescence that delayed sexual outlet began before the introduction of reliable woman-controlled contraception, but the process was hastened by the availability of contraception. Barriers to heterosexual intimacy are less formidable in an era of diminished paternal authority, so that less of the adolescent's energy must be used to break them down.

The delay in aggressive outlet which has characterized adolescence is also in a process of change, but that change is toward making permanent the inhibition of aggression. War has virtually ceased to be a viable economic alternative. Individualistic aggressive display disrupts a complex society more than a simple one. Overstimulation of aggressive drives during latency through television may lead to an overcompensatory inhibition of those drives.

The delay in autonomy imposed by traditional adolescence has diminished in some ways and intensified in others. Adolescents are less and less considered by adult society as a national resource to be protected and are thus included earlier as voters and drinkers. On the other hand, models of adult autonomy are harder for adolescents to find than formerly, since standards of adult autonomy have been modified by needs for conformity as a guarantor of security.

Facilitating and hastening the decline of adolescence as a system are the intrafamilial effects of the increasing complexity of technical problems and the consequent dehumanization of the solutional processes. A decline in male adult authority levels has accompanied the loss of economic viability in the small owner-run enterprise and the diminution of obligatory, safe, gender-distinguished roles of social conduct. There has been a compensatory decrease in female submissiveness, without, at least up to this time, an increase in female adult authority level in the society as a whole. Traditional male-oriented roles of personal autonomy based on skill are, thus, less positively coded, while successful interpersonal adaptation is more highly stressed.

The peer group has become a more important psychological support system for the adolescent in recent decades, not only because generationally transferable lessons are fewer, but also because the peer group is a valid preparation ground for the increased extensiveness of the new social systems of adulthood. The obsessive idealism peculiar to adolescence is heightened and made more important as a security giver in an adolescent population which has known less certainty in their childhoods; for that reason polar and rigid peer-supported certainty-laced positions become more attractive, whether they be political, related to drugs, religion, sex, or rebellion against adult authority. These idealisms often fail to supply lasting internal security. When they fail, the adolescent often loses peer group protection against demoralization and lapses into a detached, mildly hyperactive affect-poor state that is characterized by low attention span, restlessness and use of material objects as temporary appeasers. This detached state, often referred to as *anomie,* is in our time a frequent adolescent malady; it carries a grave personal and social prognosis.

FROM CHILDHOOD TO ADOLESCENCE

Children arrive at puberty with a different set of securities and a different set of problems than did their grandparents. Values are less forcefully inculcated in the preadolescent child because the parents are less sure of the usefulness of many traditional value systems than were their parents and grandparents. Acquisition of concrete skills, whether cognitive or manual, is less advanced in children at puberty than was true half a century ago, largely because of the effect of high density information flow in changing what is felt to be important from memorized or computational information to skills in processing information. The decline in the SAT college board scores since 1947 witnesses this trend, as does changed curricular emphasis in the schools. But the prepubertal child achieves greatest security through concrete skill acquisition. Abstract thinking is not done well before adolescence. The recent diminution in value solidity and concrete skill solidity among latency-age children reduces their readiness for the new stresses brought by puberty and its aftermaths.

In these times the child fears father less because father has less authority and is less rigid in his behavioral styles toward the child. The child adores mother less because mother has been removed from her shell of self-abasing reliance and reliability. Issues of shared autonomy and parallelisms of behaviors have replaced those of balanced needs and complementarities for most American couples. Deprived of consensually validated systems of complementarity, the American marriage has to adopt to more here-and-now conflictual issues and create a dynamic of adaptation—or else fail. To the child this change allows greater participation. There are fewer (in the view of many of us too few) areas of "you're not old enough to know" for the child. The attention that the child gives to emotional issues between the parents on an overt level is thus heightened. The easy acceptance of the traditional reliant and partly helpless role by the child is lessened.

Children's readiness level for adolescence has become further eroded in this generation by another set of factors. The earliest years of child development, up to about age three, are becoming more difficult for children as the nonverbal affective responses from the mother have become less bound by code and convention. Mothers have less unquestioned reliance in the appropriateness of their maternal role, the primacy of the child in their life space, and the security of the affectional and economic support system of marriage. The mother is as often as not working and, because of personal and/ or societal ambivalence toward her earner status, frequently finds it difficult to integrate her priorities of family and job, of nurturance focus and aggression focus; she is then likely to transmit frequent frustration signals to her child.

The very young child is dealing basically with questions of whether the world is a good place, whether he/she can develop usable and reliable skills which lead to pleasure rather than frustration, and whether he/she can get along as an individuated person without a kind of magic symbiotic attachment to the mother. These questions, of course, are linked to one another. There is strong clinical evidence from our adolescents, as well as from our adult patients who are currently parents, that the level of certainty and trusting reliance which a young child must achieve in order to answer those questions in a growth-oriented way is more and more often not attained. The level of reliability of pleasure outcomes is then not high enough in those earliest years, with the consequences of these failures in our adolescent and adult populations becoming increasingly frequent. These consequences include pessimism as concerns new areas of exploration or inquiry; polar images of self, with persistence of feelings of helplessness and/or omnipotence; search for absolute certainty; shallow response patterns in interpersonal relations; hyperactivity, with its accompanying loss of attention to external stimuli; and a partial failure of differentiation between positive and negative outcomes, with any outcome being coded as better than no outcome at all.

There is, further, in children lacking this basic security an expectation of frustration which becomes self-fulfilling in that they do not allow themselves to see the other as being non-frustrating. The parent who is insecure in terms of personal autonomy, disconnected from the old rules, tense about what will work, aware of opportunities but functionally unable to utilize them, transmits to the child the message "Don't ask me to be your certainty. I can't be my own. Go away and find your own answers." It is in that setting that children arrive at puberty with muted optimism in their life possibilities, wariness in terms of the role of authority in helping or harming them, and widespread but shallow emotional capacities. Not all children are beset by these problems; comparatively few children are crippled by them, but most children arriving at puberty today show stigmata of these influences to one extent or another.

WHEN DOES ADOLESCENCE END TODAY?

What kinds of events serve to end adolescence in our time, and what does today's adolescent have to look forward to? Identity formation, a coalescing of values, skills, and ambitions into a reasonably coherent and bounded self, requires a kind of optimism and solidity of values and skill security difficult for most current adolescents to attain. Insofar as entry into adulthood depends on firm identity formation, today's adolescents carry many typically adolescent attitudes into an adult chronology. The transition to adult responsibilities is used widely as a significator of adulthood. In an affluent society, this transition too is gradual. But while adulthood rites have virtually disappeared, marriage and full-time employment still have some effective role in this regard.

Once across the boundary into adulthood, young Americans can look forward to a life of enhanced options through affluence; multiple relationships; low to moderate authority; limited career aims; shared autonomy; pleasure out of a bottle, a pill, sexuality, and/or charismatic systems; guaranteed basic support systems; and relatively early growth toward acceptance of self. Some adults attempt to recreate the conditions of security and certainty in which their grandparents grew up through charismatic religion, retreat, or utopia. These efforts are often only temporarily successful because the wider society does not provide consensual validation to them.

Of course, most of these young adults will themselves become parents. Ideally, the adult parent will be able to live under conditions of some insecurity without undue anxiety and be able at the same time to impart to his/her children a sense of security so the child can have a base from which to grow, adaptively and with optimism. Having been deprived of such parenting, many of today's adolescents perceive their expected future as adults with some degree of pessimism and apprehension. How they, in turn, will do as parents is open to worrisome doubt.

Let me say one last word in this area—this one about history. None of the above trends connected to the lessening of the consensual validation of social systems will diminish in the foreseeable future. In other parts of the world, where our political and social freedoms are lacking, many systems are consensually validated, with powerful deterrents to nonconformity. The securities and certainties thus attained retard change, reduce the amount of ambiguous information flow, and tend to preserve the stable and custom-bound intrafamilial sets so favorable to early childhood development. Without some kind of affirmative actions in our society to counter the negative impacts described above, the tendency to demand security at whatever cost could become a compelling political and social factor in the United States.

SUMMARY

Societal stability and adaptiveness can only coexist when consensually validated support systems exists which encourage drive-reduction and integration of defensive systems in the children and adolescents within the society. The United States currently is in the grip of historical, cultural, and psychological forces which lead our young people in the opposite direction, as argued above. Our efforts must be to reverse the resultant negative trends in our adolescent population to avoid anomie, narcissism, frantic and often extremist obsessive idealism, detachment and isolation.

Our task as professionals is to upgrade our skills, our sensitivities, our understanding of the adolescent population, so that we can be effective in helping the adolescent to an identity integration and a free life beyond.

2

The Three Stages of Adolescence

EVERETT DULIT, M.D., PH.D.

This chapter has as its goal the setting down of an overview of principal themes and issues in normal adolescent development to serve as framework, context, foundation and backdrop against which to set the more detailed material concerning pathology and treatment that will unfold in the course of this text as the subject is progressively developed. I propose to do that by surveying the second decade of life, that fateful stretch of years, from three points of view. First of all is the perspective of *sheer description,* capturing psychological reality live, like the good novelist or filmmaker. Call that the naturalistic or phenomenological approach—ground to which I find myself returning again and again in my work, ground far closer to the heart of good thinking and of good science than one might think from the way in which one sees clinicians abandoning it so regularly for the presumably higher ground of formulations and language more abstract and more theoretical. In my own view, the reverse is true. It is hard to beat a good description (it is hard to achieve one also). Speaking for myself, I tend to see the ring of truth-in-description as the very foundation of our work and even of our skills. To get it just right—what it's like to be the particular person we're working with—that's the key. We need to feel it and to be able to say it in words—in words for ourselves, in words for them. With one's eye on that from beginning to end, the work tends to go well no matter what. When one gets too far away from that, it seems to me to go not so well no matter what.

13

Yet one does want ideas and principles and more abstract truths, so my second pass over the same decade will be from the point of view of the *key organizing principles and concepts of psychoanalytic developmental thinking,* and the shifting balance through adolescence among the inner agencies and forces and groupings of psychological functions which analytic theory emphasizes. And, finally, I will make a third pass over the same terrain, seen from yet a third vantage point, this time emphasizing key themes drawn from the study of the *development of intelligence*—cognitive development à la Piaget. Along the way, there will be some questions raised, some qualifications required, some revisions introduced by important work done in our time, and towards the end some gratuitous commentary on themes of special interest to me.

DESCRIPTION OF NORMAL ADOLESCENCE

Let us begin with the descriptive level. Adolescence has a rather well-defined beginning and a rather ill-defined ending. The beginning is marked by the biological event of puberty. Indeed, if one were to seek but a single concept in terms of which to define adolescence, one could catch a lion's share of the truth by speaking of adolescence as the human psychological response to the impact of the fateful biological event of puberty, that response set within and powerfully shaped by the context of family, culture and subculture. Puberty can be seen as a biological gauntlet thrown down by nature, a shock wave, hitting like a ton of bricks, at first powerfully unsettling, the initial impact followed by tremors, reverberations and repercussions, only gradually settling down. This is one view of the matter, representing the adolescent as victim, and then survivor, of an upheaval from within which mercifully then subsides on its own. There is much truth to that. Or one could take another view, one giving a more active role to the adolescent, those reverberations seen as settling down *because* of psychological work done and progressive mastery of the impact of puberty, puberty conceptualized thereby more as challenge, the adolescent seen less as victim and more as hero and doer, as catcher and tamer of thunderbolts from within— also much truth to that. And all of that is set within and profoundly shaped by social-cultural forces and, in particular, by the family, partly mediator of the culture to the child, and partly a system uniquely itself, a deeply formative psychological surround, a kind of a womb, a kind of a foundry, within which the child—to become adolescent to become adult—is warmed and cooled and heated and tempered and hammered (sometimes hammering back to be sure) conned and cajoled and loved and hated and influenced into some kind of shape and finally born out of the family, into the outside world.

The ending of adolescence is ill-defined in nature. Some interfaces in nature are like that: without a sharp demarcation—the fading of light towards the end of day or the edge of the mist. Adolescence just shades off gradually into young adulthood. The reasons for that are not difficult to specify. Many of the features that define adolescence persist into young adulthood, as psychological currents that flow together with and are integrated into other currents coming to the fore in the twenties, thus only gradually losing the defining prominence they had in adolescence. The sheer intensity of feeling tone characteristic of adolescence could serve as a good example; it is certainly present in young adulthood and can certainly be part of varieties of normal later adulthood, but integrated, flowing together with and moderated by capacities for restraint and acceptance, forbearance and perspective—human psychological potentialities which are not so likely to be fully developed in adolescence (even in the best of adolescence) as they can become in adulthood.

A second determinant of the gradualness to the end of adolescence is that there are a number of *separate* psychological currents running, in combination, to give to adolescence its characteristic coloration. But they don't all shift over into their adult forms, so to speak, simultaneously. Some shift sooner, some later, and with much individual variation. Hence, there is a gradual ending *in nature,* not something that "further research will clarify" (that phrase a reflex tic of our times and field that has begun to make me wince). Some realities don't have sharp edges. Obsessionals and researchers may not like that. I rather do. Sometimes soft focus *is* reality in life, especially in clinical work.

But even with that inherent imprecision about endpoint, one can observe and speak of a rather wide range of variations in the duration of adolescence. Depending on the combined influence of socio-cultural context, family dynamics and intrapsychic determinants, one can see an adolescence varying in duration from the one extreme of a process virtually compressed, so to speak, into the single brief rite de passage that one sometimes sees in the primitive tribal society, through the intermediate durations of less than a decade character-istic of adolescence in an agrarian society or of some varieties of working-class adolescence in our own society, all the way over to the more prolonged forms of adolescence lasting a decade or more typical for the educated middle-class youngster in Westernized cultures like our own, or lasting even into the late twenties for a certain kind of nonpathological young adult pursuing complex psychosocial goals and his own inner relation to those goals, that kind of young adult-hood described in the work of Kenneth Keniston and said by him to be increasingly emergent in our affluent times. That kind of "adolescence" is similar to a kind of "not-quite-adolescence-but-not-quite-adulthood" with which we have long been familiar as a "stage" (or style) of life lasting into the late twenties in graduate students, or even into the late thirties in those who pursue advanced training or apprenticeship roles which long defer "full" adult professional roles—the psychoanalytic candidate or the assistant professor, for example. (I remember a respected teacher of mine, an adolescent psychiatrist, with many of the key themes of adolescence very much alive and writ large within himself. When I was his student he used to like to say that adolescence normally runs into the forties. As we've both grown older, I notice of late he says fifties.)

And, finally, on this point the reader is asked to consider the thought that just as richly flavored soup generally requires long slow simmering on the stove, and just as fine wines generally require a longer time in the bottle, so also does it seem to many of us who work in this area that the more richly developed kinds of adulthood seem generally to be preceded by the longer kinds of adolescence, by a decade or more of simmering and ripening, in what can thus be identified as a necessary prelude to a more fully developed adult-hood. That is a point about which there is room for an honest difference of opinion and on which it would be well to get more data before speaking with confidence. But it is probably a valid perspec-tive, and if so, rich with implications for the work that we do with young people, particularly those young people where culture, family or the adolescent moves to close off those psychological epiphyses prematurely.

THE THREE STAGES OF ADOLESCENCE

It says in the Haggadah, that ancient text read aloud by Jews the world over on Passover, that whosoever doth not make mention that night of three things will not be considered worthy. For that occasion they are the unleavened bread, the bitter herbs, and the Paschal lamb, all meaningful symbols within the ceremony. For an adolescent psychiatrist on the subject of adolescent development, the three things are: early adolescence, middle adolescence and late adolescence. No adolescent psychiatrist worth his salt fails to make those distinctions or some equivalent. For someone absorbed in work with this age group, given the rapid rate of change from 12 through 20, the term "adolescent" is just too broad, too global, too overinclusive. That tripartite division—early/middle/late—or something like it, becomes necessary, emerges quite naturally, and begins to come as second nature to anyone really absorbed in the work. Early, middle, late—those are categories certainly not sharply defined at the edges, definitely overlapping and shading off, each into the next, but each having a distinctly different center, each having a recognizably different central theme.

Early is 12, 13, 14—the junior high school years. Middle is 14, 15, 16, 17—the high school years. Late is 17, 18, 19, 20, shading off into young adulthood. What are the central themes and the characteristic picture for each stage?

Early Adolescence

Early adolescence, a year or two after the onset of puberty, and maybe even just a bit before as the biological storm begins to gather momentum, is a time of great emotional lability. It is time of normal abnormality, of normal insanity—the junior high school years. Nobody wants to work in junior high school—and for good reason. It's a madhouse. For most youngsters, the relative calm and order of the latency years are shattered by the impact of puberty. Even the vitality of childhood, shot through with good feelings bubbling up, changes its character upon coming into early adolescence, becoming more tense and intense, more frantic and frenetic, edgy, with the quality of inner turmoil and strong feelings barely held in check, under strain, regularly bursting through and spilling over. These are years of tears and tantrums for no reason at all, of overreactions and rushing off in a huff, of mysterious moods understood by no one—not by parents, teachers, therapists, and least of all by the youngsters themselves. Emotions run rampant. Unpredictability is the rule. Frank cruelty is distressingly commonplace (*Lord of the Flies* variety), a major recurrent problem in any junior high school. In the suburbs, most often, it is psychological cruelty of a sort rarely seen in elementary school or high school. Sometimes it is physical cruelty, which is not at all uncommon in the ghetto. (Most of those kids who kill and torture captives from the other gang in the real ghetto are 13 and 14, not late adolescents like in *West Side Story*.)

In some critical respects, the young adolescent is the quintessential adolescent, problematic, very much betwixt and between, between the calm of latency and the calmer waters of middle adolescence yet to come, neither here nor there, unsettled, in turmoil. This is probably the region on the age range from zero through adulthood most difficult to work with in therapy. There's an aphorism within the field of adolescent therapy (and I don't mean among therapists who don't work with adolescents, but among those of us who do) that the best thing to do with a young adolescent is to put him on a waiting list until he is a middle adolescent. That's only a quip, but it is quip that's trying to tell us something. If you find it difficult to work with young adolescents, you are not alone!

Middle Adolescence

Then comes the years of middle adolescence: 15, 16, 17—roughly speaking, the high school years. Middle adolescence sees a distinct settling down, a noticeably greater capacity for composure and compromise, a way of relating to adults that is more complex and more civilized, a greater capacity for grace and empathy, and the by no means insignificant arrival of an advancing capacity for deception. The middle adolescent is better able to think one thing and say another and carry it off as a successful performance, not ordinarily regarded as a worthy milestone in human development. But maybe it should be. It is a real *cognitive* achievement, a near neighbor to and even a necessary ingredient to civilized behavior. The greater civility of middle adolescence is, in any event, a welcome arrival. Also, by middle adolescence the intense self-absorption of early adolescence begins to subside somewhat and to be replaced, as it were, by a greater capacity again to become absorbed in work, a shift back to the rather more favorable balance, in that respect, that prevailed during latency.

Further, the defensively charged total commitment to the peer group, "my peer group right or wrong," so typical of the early adolescent, begins to give way to a rather more differentiated response. The young person is much better able to stand separate from the group when necessary, to recognize the people in the peer group or the trends in the peer group that it would be better to avoid, and to recognize the need to protect himself or herself from those people and those trends. He begins to have the social skills necessary to carry this off without looking too clumsy or "chicken" in the process, and to have the strength necessary to stick to his own best interests even when he does get some flack for it.

Another observable feature of the transition from early to middle adolescence—a small point but one that for me conveys rather nicely the change in dominant emotional tone—is to compare and contrast the feeling tone (the "vibes") at parties where the kids are junior high school age versus high school age parties. For the young adolescent, a party is usually a pretty tough time for all concerned, with so much stridency, strain and tension shot through the allegedly "good time" as to make the sensitive observer fairly cringe. Whereas, even at their most rambunctious, a bunch of reasonably "together" high school kids at a party really seem to be able to have a genuine good time, giving off the sound of genuine good cheer. One just does not hear that sound very often at junior high school parties. Overall, it becomes easier to live with middle adolescents and easier to work things out with them, at home, at school and in therapy. Not easy—but easier.

Late Adolescence

Finally, standing on that more secure platform of middle adolescence, the young person begins reaching, as he or she moves into and through adolescence, for progressively more complex levels of "getting himself or herself together," a phrase of our time rather nicely evocative of a central ask for the age, perhaps *the* central psychological task for the age: *identity formation.* That is a concept, of course, contributed and elaborated principally by Erik Erikson (1956), who has cast a strong light on the importance in late adolescence of the psychological work of weaving together into one fabric, of synthesizing into one relatively unique, relatively coherent good enough psychological self and sense of self, all the diverse strands of constitutional givens, favored capacities, progressively forming character traits, favorite defensive constellations, partial identifications, and chosen roles that have been spun out by the developmental process through the years of childhood and early/ middle adolescence. This is work done in late adolescence. This is the time when major life choices concerning work and career begin to be made. The exploratory experimental trying-things-on-for-size quality normally present and even necessary to some degree in middle adolescence begins to give way to more definite "choices" and to the increasingly irreversible emergence by late adolescence and young adulthood of the kind of person one is going to be. As Pumpian-Mindlin (1965) has written, middle adolescence is a time of omnipotentiality, a time during which, in some real sense, "all things" (i.e. many choices) are possible, especially under optimal circumstances of development. But late adolescence is a time of closing doors, of going one way and not the other. It would be difficult to improve on the beautiful expression of that in the poem by Robert Frost. Selecting lines taken from "The Road Not Taken"*:

> *Two roads diverged in a yellow wood,*
> *And sorry I could not travel both*
> *And be one traveler, long I stood*
> *And looked down one as far as I could*
> *To where it bent in the undergrowth;*
>
> *Then took the other, as just as fair,*
> *And having perhaps the better claim.*

> *I shall be telling this with a sigh*
> *Somewhere ages and ages hence:*
> *Two roads diverged in a wood, and I—*
> *I took the one less traveled by,*
> *And that has made all the difference.*

"The one less traveled by" is an important theme in the poem, and also in adolescent development. But even more important is the central theme of *choice*, of *having* to choose, and the sense *while* choosing that one will be looking back "ages and ages hence" on a choice that will have "made all the difference."

PSYCHOANALYTIC PERSPECTIVES ON ADOLESCENCE

Let us sample now the psychoanalytic stream of ideas about adolescence—a body of work and an intellectual current that has set some of the key terms within which we think in these times, and a perspective which serves many of us in the field at the very least as a kind of basic point of departure, for agreement, partial agreement or even substantial disagreement. Principal early contributors have been Sigmund Freud (1905), Anna Freud (1958), Peter Blos (1962), Kurt Eissler (1950), Leo Spiegel (1951, 1958), Helene Deutsch (1944, 1945, 1969), Erik Erikson (1956) and others. A central organizing feature of the psychoanalytic point of view is the attention it pays to the interactions among three principal clusters of mental functions, definitions by now part of the familiar terminology of our times: the concept of *id* grouping the more primitive, childlike, impulsive, body-oriented mental functions; the concept of *ego* grouping the more mature, executive, coping, mastering, reality-oriented, inner-regulating functions; the concept of *superego* grouping an uneasy mix of mental functions all having something to do with right or wrong, shalt or shalt not, varying in tone from the most harsh, primitive, fanatic quality of id at its worst all the way over to the most mature, thoughtful, judicious and wise quality of ego at its best.

Let us concentrate for a moment on the *balance of forces* between ego and id as we move from childhood through adolescence. The years of early childhood, the magic years, to use Selma Fraiberg's felicitous phrase, are given their characteristic coloration by id forces.

Almost by definition, id is childlike. By latency the balance has shifted. To use the Freudian metaphor of horse and rider, ego is in the saddle, id reined in and under control. The fires become relatively banked, leaving latency dominated by a quality of relative moderation, propriety and order: a place for everything and everything in its place, family gatherings and family outings, every state with its own capitol, every country with its own product, every word with its own spelling, every question with an answer—an obsessional's delight. Or to put it more kindly and equally truly, it is a good time of life for the good boy and the good girl and the good parent.

And then the inner storm gathers force and explodes and everything comes unstuck. The horse bolts. Id is off again and running, with sexual and aggressive forces riding the crest of a wave of hormones. Ego is thrown from the saddle and left running along behind, a poor second, unceremoniously unseated, government once again in the hands of the extremists. And as a consequence of that restoration of id domination we see in the years of early adolescence a recapitulation at many levels of some of the qualities of early childhood, a regressive pull, with the young adolescent regularly overcome by and wallowing in the wash of it, with classes in junior high school regularly being broken up by giggling fits and funny noises, and giggling fits about funny noises.

In some respects this is a regression to the stormy pregenital years, the years before latency. But in one very important respect it is significantly different. Now that whole complex of aggressive and sexual feelings is set in a body increasingly approximating (indeed becoming) an adult body, increasingly muscular, increasingly erotic, increasingly able really "to do it." That is a powerful psychological reality, perceived at some level by all concerned, and reacted to notably by the adolescent's putting distance between self and parents —real distance (behind locked doors and out of the house) and, above all, psychological distance. And to make matters worse, this whole configuration of emotional upheaval and defensive counter-reactions comes at a bad moment in the course of parallel independent developments in the cognitive realm, at just the time when cognitive structures are undergoing a major overhaul of their own in the course of their transition from concrete to formal patterns of organization. Thus a major component of the defensive system (i.e., cognition, thinking) is in a state of renovation and instability just when the tidal waves strike. This is bad timing on the part of nature, leading to a bad time for all concerned—for parents, for therapists, and mostly for the adolescents themselves.

But there are at least two saving graces to early adolescence. First, as Blos and others have emphasized, that very same fluidity that gives to early adolescence its runny quality (and which often makes therapy at this age seem rather like building structures in the sand at the edge of the waves) also has a fateful potential for good, because along with everything else that becomes a bit runny in the heat of adolescence so do some of the not-so-satisfactory defensive constellations laid down in childhood, those not-so-satisfactory resolutions of infantile and childhood conflicts of the sort that tend to be at the core of the neurotic process. Adolescence thus offers a potential second chance, an important new opportunity for doing a better job of conflict resolution this second time around, working now with the emerging more mature resources and cognitive capacities of middle and late adolescence. The second (and only other) saving grace of early adolescence is that it ends.

In summary, then, key elements of the psychoanalytic view are a surge of sexual and aggressive forces carried on the crest of the wave of hormones striking in puberty, constituting an assault of id on ego, with ego relatively overcome, even in rout, with psychic structure softening in the "heat" and becoming disorganized, with an upsurge of inner turmoil, some of it manifest, some of it latent. Yet, on the positive side, there exists a valuable second chance, while the substance of the psychic structure is still molten, for revision of some not-so-good defensive patterns that were laid down in childhood. Middle adolescence is thus perhaps one optimal time for that kind of psychic reshaping. In therapy, that means the opportunity for working with a mind appreciably more mature than the child's mind and with a psychic structure that is beginning to cool off enough to hold new shape, but not yet set, as it *does* tend to become, for better and/or worse by late adolescence, into the characterological forms, wonderful or not so wonderful, neurotic or not so neurotic, that are likely to endure as basic patterns in that person for the remainder of life.

Some Newer Perspectives

Does it really work out that way? Does the psychoanalytic formulation just outlined truly capture reality? Well, as with virtually any of the best of our efforts to contain the complexity of human behavior within the bounds of a fairly brief formulation, the answer has to be "yes and no." The author believes that the classical psychoanalytic formulation does indeed provide a solid foundation upon which one can really stand. But it is a foundation upon which one must also build qualifications, caveats and supplements. Some of them have been provided by important work done in the last decade, including notably the work of Daniel Offer (see Chapter 4) and the work of James Masterson, particularly the follow-up study published about 10 years ago under the title *The Psychiatric Dilemma of Adolescence.*

Offer, studying the development over time of a sizable group of normal adolescent boys, brings to our attention compelling data showing that manifest turmoil of the sort that would be the fully direct expression of the psychoanalytic perspectives just outlined seems present strikingly and unmistakably in only about one-fifth of his sample, a modest to moderate percentage. Furthermore, an almost equally large group showed outwardly virtually none of that, coasting through adolescence mostly with "a smoothness of purpose and a self-assurance of their progression toward a meaningful and fulfilling adult life." There is also a rather larger group, approximately 40% of the total sample, that showed a pattern of developmental spurts separated by periods of stasis, with manifest turmoil and anxiety in surges, and intervals of blocking, overcontrol, depression and shaky self-esteem.

Although Offer's work has been represented by some as contradicting the basic psychoanalytic concept of the surge of inner forces and the presence of inner tumult as defining and regular features of adolescence, I myself would read the data as fundamentally in support of that basic formulation but containing implications that certainly call for important qualifications and additions. Offer's data, in my reading, are basically a testimonial to the power of the *normal adolescent ego,* our best ally in the work we do daily, to keep much of outward behavior and even some of "inner behavior" under control in normal youngsters *despite* the turmoil and renovation at the core, rather like the gyrostabilizer of a ship on stormy seas— in this case inner seas. But Offer's work certainly does drive us to a more sophisticated view of adolescence than the simplest interpretations present in the early literature which suggested that manifest outward turmoil, even approaching psychotic proportions, was virtually always present and even an essential feature of normal adolescence. That is much too simple a view and is in that sense false.

The work of James Masterson extends and nicely complicates (i.e. opens up) the picture still further. In his follow-up study of 101 manifestly troubled youngsters brought for treatment to the Psychiatric Service at Payne Whitney Clinic in New York, he found that the percentage that remained impaired five or more years later (with or without treatment) was in the range of 60% overall, as high as 75% for those diagnosed personality disorder, and as high as 100% for those diagnosed sociopath. Masterson's findings, therefore, stand as a serious challenge to the reassuring notion introduced in the early literature that one didn't have to worry about most manifest turmoil in adolescence because it was, after all, just a troublesome phase of basically normal development and that "they'd grow out of it." The author's reading of Masterson's work, quite consistent with Masterson's own interpretation, would be that for those adolescents *brought for treatment* to a hospital or clinic, the odds are that the trouble is not so benign in prognosis, and that very likely they won't "just grow out of it." More likely, what they "have" is psychopathology and not just a somewhat more florid version of normal adolescent turmoil. Always there is some uncertainty in making these assessments but, if you are the betting kind, if the adolescent is actually brought to a clinic or hospital, bet on psychopathology and you'll make money. In outpatient work, probably the odds are more evenly balanced, or maybe even tipped the other way.

The author's own overview of the net effect of the revisions rightly introduced by the newer work is that, contrary to what some commentators seem to believe, or would like to believe, this newer work does *not* tell us so much what we *are* seeing when we see a troubled adolescent in our office, but rather has the virtue of making us less sure, and thus forcing us to look more sharply and more deeply.

The truth is probably most nearly served by emphasizing that one sees *everything*. One sees kids in major turmoil where that turmoil is a normal and productive part of the struggle to shape a good life and where they *make it*. One sees cases in similar turmoil where they do not make it, because they give up or are working against external odds that are too great. One sees kids in whom there is major turmoil which eventually proves to be (and may even be recognized at the outset to be) major psychopathology. One sees kids who coast through adolescence smoothly *because* they have the very best of shock absorbers and gyrostabilizers buffering them against the many jolts from a simultaneously active and even tumultuous inner emotional life. And one sees kids who coast through smoothly only by paying a very high price in rigidity and inhibition and unfulfilled human potentials, with an inhibited inner emotional life. And one sees all shades of gray in between.

All of these possibilities are present "in nature." One sees them all. Nor is any one of those categories statistically so predominant that one could reliably bet on it over its externally similar partner. For example, observed external turmoil could reflect "merely" normal adolescent turmoil or definite psychopathology. Likewise, the calm course through adolescence could equally reflect overcontrol or successful active mastery. How can one tell the difference? Does modern work provide us with reliable criteria? Yes, to some degree. But mostly the criteria are the obvious and relatively straightforward ones we use all the time in good clinical work. To recount them in detail would be co-extensive with the entirety of what this volume aspires to accomplish and certainly would exceed the bounds of this single chapter. Perhaps suffice it to say that they would include: some assessment of mastery of the various psychological tasks of adolescence, of effective coping capacities, of adequacy of object relations within the family and outside of the family, of capacity for affect control within the normal range, of the absence of major or appreciable symptomatology, of effective and satisfying involvement in learning, of a basic standard of psychological organization and no major disorganization, and other such considerations.

The trouble is that although such criteria help greatly with an appreciable proportion of the cases we see for assessment, there remains a steady and appreciable stream of cases in the hazy gray area between normally troubled adolescence and definitely pathological adolescence. In this author's opinion, even the best of our clinical criteria leave us still quite uncertain in *those* "gray area cases," which is where questions most often arise. How then *does* one make such assessments? In particular, how *does* one decide whether or not to recommend treatment? One obvious response, and, in my opinion, a very correct one would be: "By looking at the *overall* picture." All right then, you may well reply, how does one tell an "overall picture" that needs treatment from one that doesn't? That puts the question in a form I very much like. But let's put off trying to answer it to the end of this chapter and turn instead at this point to a final broad sweep over the years of adolescence, this time from the vantage point of the study of cognitive development.

COGNITIVE DEVELOPMENT IN ADOLESCENCE

The principal architect in our time, and probably for some time to come, of the basic ideas in the area of cognitive development is Jean Piaget, whose work has been a special interest area of mine. The focus here is on the thought process, the use of the mind in problem solving, the adaptive use of the mind to map and master and make sense of and, thus, more effectively to cope with the outside world. The focus here is on thinking, setting aside, for the time being, feelings and motivations. Both of those surely do play upon and relate to the thought process in a myriad of ways. But to gain focus and clarity, the cognitive approach at the outset basically sweeps those aside, lending to Piagetian perspectives a certain clear, pure, pristine, rarified quality, rather like the high mountain air of Switzerland where the principal architect of this point of view was born and has elaborated his monumental body of work and theory.

Data here are elicited by presenting the child or adolescent with a by-now-familiar repertoire of wonderfully ingenious methods and stratagems, essentially problems and challenges that set the child to thinking, followed by an open-ended "clinical interview" intended to try to get at the nature of the thought process which lies behind the child's answers. Out of decades of work with that approach has emerged the concept of a hierarchical succession of stages in the development of intelligence from childhood through adolescence into adulthood, each stage a kind of world view, each a successively perience "out there." Our focus here will be on the transition from the stage of concrete thought characteristic of the years seven through 11 into the stage of formal or abstract thought characteristic of the years of adolescence and thereafter.

What are the central themes of the concrete stage of thought? In Piaget's terminology (Piaget and Inhelder, 1958) the central themes are *The Logic of Class* and *The Logic of Relations*. The Logic of Class means that thinking is cast in terms of categories, in terms of whether something is or is not a member of a given class, those classes given by school, culture, family, but also eagerly sought by the child prepared and very ready to think in those terms, who warms to that whole game of classification and to that whole world-view. The Logic of Relations is essentially the capacity to set things into a graded ordered series, from smallest, to large, larger, largest, in size place. To this is added one-to-one correspondence, which means setting one series into correspondence with another (e.g. the bigger, the heavier). Out of those simple elements you can already see the beginnings of a kind of cause and effect paradigm (the more this *then* the more that) and of a reaching for inner invariants (for example, "the bigger, the heavier" leading on quite naturally to the concept of density). But, basically, we have, in childhood thinking, a very concrete world of categories and series, of boxes and lineups.

Then comes age 11, 12, 13 and we see the transition, at first gradual, and then, for some, with a rush, into the formal stage of thought, abstract thought à la Piaget, which replaces the orderly but limited "earthbound" quality of categorical concrete thinking. We see the emergence of thinking with a different pattern, a different structure, far more powerful and comprehensive, overarching and unencumbered. The stage of abstract thought brings the capacity to order and process complex data by utilizing patterns of organization far more complex than those of the concrete stage. It also brings the capacity to leap with the mind into untracked cognitive terrain, cognitive terra incognita, to travel in inner space, and out, to everywhere and anywhere, flying with the mind.

In Piagetian terms, at the core of that transformation lies the emergence of a structure in the mind capable of organizing in a logically meaningful way *all* of the possible states inherent in and implied by the situation at hand. Abstracting from the system at more complex way of actively organizing the Rorschach blot of ex-hand all the relevant variables and running them systematically through all their possible values, one generates a structure, a matrix in the mind that contains implicitly all possible states of the particular system at hand. Thinking in the formal abstract stage is conceptualized as having access to that matrix, and being able to move freely about within it, relating various possible states of the system at hand to one another and to the real world in ways that are equivalent to the classical logical operations, such as implication, exclusion, hypothesis, proof and disproof. The adolescent mind now begins to function as a new kind of logical machine, a tester of hypotheses, and acquires now for the first time the critically important new capacity to generate possibilities *never before actualized* in the child's experience, generated now not by memory but by *thinking,* by sheer combination and recombination of those parameters abstracted from the real world. Thus, the formal stage thinker generates *out of the mind* possibilities never before actually experienced. A classic example would be the valedictory address about "What could be but is not." The newly acquired capacity for that level of cognition is a defining characteristic of the formal stage.

It also becomes possible at this stage to begin to conceptualize things that can be thought about but that *never could be* actualized in the real world. For example, in mathematics, one can generalize from the two-dimensional world of the plane and the three-dimensional world of the solid up and out to the four-dimensional world of relativity theory, and on to the n-dimensional world of modern algebra. The three-dimensional world? "Oh yes, that's where I happen to live," says the abstract thinker, "a mere special case," like happening to live in New York City, or Washington. Abstract thought brings such a new capacity for the soaring overarching perspective, as clearly to constitute one major root (the *cognitive* root) of the familiar grandiosity of adolescence, expressing itself in forms that run the gamut from adolescent idealism to adolescent delinquency.

Thus, going from the concrete stage to the formal, we observe a major reversal of priorities—possibility now coming to dominate over actuality, with the full range of possibilities inherent in the situation now generated strictly by the mind—a heady experience (pun intended). We observe the capacity now to think not only about things, but about thoughts, about propositions, hypotheses, ideas, ideologies, abstractions, truth, beauty, sunset, justice, an almost awesome opening up of horizons, enormously engaging for some—for others, frightening or avoided, or derogated or not their cup of tea. For others, it is a terrain into which they rush and become confused. Sometimes such confusion is soft psychopathology and just a casualty of newfound cognitive capacities not yet integrated and tamed. Sometimes it is the outer form of severe, biologically based psychopathological thought disorder. The distinction is sometimes difficult to make, even for the experienced observer. More often, it is *not* so difficult.

Although almost all individuals pass through the earlier Piagetian stages, only about one-third of the normal population moves fully into this stage of formal thought and makes of it a meaningful effective part of their lives. Thus, formal stage functioning has something of the quality of an achievement. It is, thus, something midway between such special talents as mathematical or musical or graphical talents (which are even less common—achieved by just a few percent of the population, depending on how stringent one is in criteria) and the cognitive achievements of the earlier Piagetian stages (which are relatively universal in educated Westernized groups). That makes the formal stage a kind of cognitive maturity which, like other forms of psychological maturity and the other developmental landmarks of later life, adolescence included, is only partially attained by most and appreciably attained only by some.

Then, in late adolescence, come further critical developments, some young adults repudiating all of those potentials for abstract thought as kid stuff, literally and figuratively storing their poems in the attic, and settling down to job, payroll, mortgage, insurance, family, kids and that kind of reality: the butcher, the baker, the candlestick maker. And then there are others, those who aspire to be mindworkers (you and me?), who work to weave those capacities for high-flying abstraction together with self-critical earth-rooted reality-testing elements, mined elsewhere, forging those two capacities together into an alloy stronger than either one alone, into a thought process that will combine the freedom and the power of the former with the substance and the solidity of the latter—psychological work done very actively in young adulthood—and thereafter.

OTHER PERSPECTIVES

The material up to this point in the chapter has been intended as an overview of key themes and perspectives in normal adolescent development, but as is invariably the case in any brief survey, some very important special perspectives have gone altogether unremarked. It seems prudent at this point at least to touch on some of them, even if only in the form of topic headings. Virtually nothing has been mentioned in this chapter about the highly important subject of sexual behavior, about masturbation, the beginnings of sexual intimacy, about the wide range of normal patterns, about the social side of sexual behavior, and about changing patterns in our time, as well as parental reactions to those changes. Happily, some of those themes are developed in other chapters in this text. In like manner, this chapter might well have included some elaboration of the approach to describing normal development which speaks in terms of the psychological *tasks* of each stage of life. Some principal examples for adolescence would be: mastery of the sexual and aggressive surges of adolescence; mastery of dependency-independency issues, moving out of the family and into the outside world, identity formation; and coping with the very special narcissistic developmental issues that come to the fore in adolescence (finding some middle course between grandiosity and the complete loss of the sense of being "special" and valued that most children do get to some degree in most "good enough" families but which is increasingly at risk with increasingly unprotected exposure to an outside world that clearly doesn't feel that way about you at all).

This chapter might well have spoken of the development of cognitive potential as task, or of the development of skills and talents, a very practical matter that psychotherapists can easily set aside as business for the teacher or others. But adolescence is a critical period for the development of many skills and talents, often without the possibility of a later second chance. The more my own adolescent patients of a decade or more ago move into and through their twenties and I see how severely it limits options to be without special skills, the more seriously do I take the job of helping the patients I have now to take seriously the importance of developing skills and talents, and of mastering the conflicts that interfere, so that they can become *somebody* who can do something well.

And, finally, that line of thought leads back to the question I left in the air midway through. To do that kind of work one has to be making assessments, all the time, of young lives in transition, and of how they're going, and of when is it "good enough" to "leave it be" and when is it not. How does one make such assessments of young lives in progress? When such a unique and complex pattern of psychological organization/disorganization as a troubled adolescent comes into one's purview, and he or she isn't obviously wonderful or obviously disturbed but a little bit of each, how does one size up what's going on and how to try to proceed? Well, the answer I would (and will) give to that very real question which confronts us daily as we do our work is an answer that will run counter to trends towards "science" and measurement running so strongly in our field just now. I am well aware that there are many good and excellent people, some of them contributors to this volume, who would strongly differ with the point of view for which I want here to be a voice. But there are some of you to whom what I write will be congenial because it will echo trends in your own line of thought about these matters. It is to you that I address myself. (We've got to stick together, to encourage each other.)

When I think about what I do in my daily work of assessing how things are going in the lives of the adolescents with whom I work every day in my office or in the hospital, it seems to me that what I am doing is more nearly captured by metaphors and language from the field of esthetics than by metaphors and language from the field of science. When we are assessing young lives in progress, we are confronting highly complex patterns of psychological organization shifting in time. Making such assessments, in my opinion, is work that is not so much like what is ordinarily meant by or ordinarily approached by scientific measurement, but much more like what a sophisticated critic does when he sizes up a book or a film or a painting, *including* that the critical work and critical product itself is usually an entity of a similarly high order of complexity, rather than, for example, being a simple number. (Note that I am *not at all* making the point here that psychological assessment and esthetics are similar because "they both deal with feelings" more than "science" does.) I am making a point here about the nature of knowledge, about epistemology, about ways of using the mind when thinking about and approaching highly complex patterns of organization changing in time where the numbers involved and the degrees of inner complexity are of an order of magnitude considerably greater than they are for the phenomena in the physical world that have been so successfully mastered and mapped by the cognitive forms we associate with the word science (let alone that what is so often called science by those eager to bring measurement oriented approaches into our field is probably closer to the language and forms of *engineering* than to the *broader* language and forms of science). Science and engineering certainly have their place as components in the clinical enterprise, but the essence of the clinical enterprise, in my opinion, is at a level of organization and numerical complexity that does not lend itself to the data-gathering and processing approach we are accustomed to associating with science and engineering. In my view, the approach to finding meaning and order in systems at this level of complexity is through language and metaphor that come closer to the language and metaphor of esthetics and criticism, a neighboring field in which the mind of man is also approaching complex patterns. There is nothing so remarkable about that if you think about it for a bit. Like the man in Moliere who was astonished, impressed and delighted that he spoke prose, good clinicians are in fact doing that all the time. The trouble comes when in search of an illusory objectivity they depart from that approach and content themselves with measurable simplicities unequal to containing the complexities that are "of the essence" in clinical work.

How does one assess an adolescent? One does it the same way a good judge of paintings and poems, and even of fine wines, does it —by first "getting under one's belt" as much knowledge and experience as one can and as much exposure to adolescents and to the work of other adolescent diagnosticians as one can, letting it all "sink in," and then, each time when confronted anew with the task of assessment, experiencing and facilitating within oneself a "rising to the surface" in a different and unpredictable way of some judgmental response which is basically within-the-discipline and yet simultaneously crucially unique. One thus becomes a kind of vehicle or agent of a process of critical appraisal and interaction that I am insisting, in its essences, does now and always will resist specification and direct transmission (though there are, to be sure, important *part* aspects of it that can be specified and directly transmitted), quite parallel to the situation that prevails and that I would insist will always prevail for other similar critical appraisals at this level of complexity. Clearly this is a line of thought about which more could be said, both pro and con, but perhaps it is best at this point to leave the pleasure of spinning out some of those implications as an exercise for the interested reader.

SUMMARY

This chapter set out to make a descriptive survey of the three stages of adolescence, followed by a second overview emphasizing psychoanalytic themes and more current revisions of same necessitated by recent work in studies of adolescence. There followed a third sweep emphasizing cognitive themes, and then respects fleetingly paid to a cluster of important special topics. Finally, I have allowed myself the pleasure of concluding with a special point of view about our work that I find intriguing, valid and useful, and that I hope some readers will as well.

REFERENCES

BLOS, P. *On Adolescence: A Psychoanalytic Interpretation.* New York: Free Press, 1962.

DEUTSCH, H. *The Psychology of Women,* I: New York: Grune & Stratton, 1944.

DEUTSCH, H. *The Psychology of Women,* II: New York: Grune & Stratton, 1945.

DEUTSCH, H. *Selected Problems of Adolescents.* New York: International Universities Press, 1969.

DULIT, E. Adolescent thinking: The formal stage. *Journal of Youth and Adolescence,* 1:281-301, 1972.

EISSLER, K. *The Psychoanalytic Study of the Child,* 5:97-121. New York: International Universities Press, 1950.

EISSLER, K. *The Psychoanalytic Study of the Child,* 13:223-54. New York: International Universities Press, 1958.

ERIKSON, E. H. The problem of ego identity. *Journal of the American Psychoanalytic Association,* 4:56-121, 1956.

FREUD, A. Adolescence, *The Psychoanalytic Study of the Child,* 13:255-278. New York: International Universities Press, 1958.

FREUD, S. (1905). Three essays on the theory of sexuality. *Standard Edition,* 7:125-245. London: Hogarth, 1953.

MASTERSON, J. F. *The Psychiatric Dilemma of Adolescence.* Boston: Little, Brown, 1967.

PIAGET, J. & INHELDER, B. *The Growth of Logical Thinking.* New York: Basic Books, 1958.

PUMPIAN-MINDLIN, E. Omnipotentiality, youth, and commitment. *Journal of American Academy of Child Psychiatry,* 4:1-18, 1965.

SPIEGEL, L. A. *The Psychoanalytic Study of the Child,* 6:375-393, New York: International Universities Press, 1951.

SPIEGEL, L. A. *The Psychoanalytic Study of the Child,* 13:296-308, New York: International Universities Press, 1958.

3
Puberty and Associated Medical Disorders of Adolescence

ROBERT B. SHEARIN, M.D.
and
RICHARD L. JONES, M.D.

The hormonal changes that occur during the process of growing from childhood to adulthood dramatically define the adolescent period from a physiological and anatomical standpoint. Health care workers must understand the basic changes that occur in order to effectively deal with adolescents. It is also necessary that they be familiar with certain medical conditions which may go unrecognized in the patient who is being followed for a psychosocial problem. In many instances, it is the psychiatrist, psychologist, social worker or nurse who recognizes a potential problem and refers the adolescent for a medical evaluation. This chapter deals with understanding the endocrinology of puberty and recognizing certain medical problems that may be present during this period of life.

ENDOCRINOLOGY OF PUBERTY

The second most significant growth period in life occurs during adolescence. It is responsible in most cases for the final 25% of linear growth and almost 50% of ideal body weight (Barnes, 1975). Inextricably linked to this physical growth are the physical and psychological changes that so characteristically mark the differences between child and adult. Care of the adolescent must be based on a

35

fundamentally sound knowledge of the normal physiological and anatomical developmental changes that occur during the growth from childhood to adolescence. With a thorough understanding of the adolescent's growth pattern and hormonal changes, health care professionals can begin to understand the alterations that occur when medical problems either change, retard, or prevent these milestones from progressing in a regular pattern.

In the United States, longitudinal and cross-sectional studies over the last hundred years have revealed an increase in height averaging one inch every 25 years for both sexes. Menarche has occurred earlier with each generation. The average adolescent will begin to menstruate during the twelfth year, almost five years sooner than adolescents did 100 years ago (Daniel, 1970). The causes for these earlier pubertal changes are multiple, but certainly nutritional, environmental and genetic factors have been of paramount importance.

Growth changes usually occur in the same sequence among adolescents, with considerable variation in the time of onset, as well as in the degree of change and in the velocity at which these changes occur (Tanner, 1962). Growth occurs in every organ system of the body, with only the thymus, tonsils, and adenoids showing an obvious decrease in size. Skeletal mass, heart, lungs, liver, spleen, kidneys, pancreas, thyroids, adrenals, gonads, phallus, and uterus all double in size, while the central nervous system increases minimally (Barnes, 1975). The onset of puberty is marked by the appearance of secondary sexual characteristics that result from the trophic effects of the gonadal hormones (i.e., estrogen and testosterone). These changes account for all future alterations that occur in the adolescent body. The endocrinology of puberty is not fully understood, but it is known that puberty is dependent on the maturation of the central nervous system and the hypothalamic-pituitary-gonadal regulatory mechanisms.

The Hypothalamic-Pituitary Axis

During childhood, the hypothalamic-pituitary axis is sensitive to feedback inhibition by small amounts of gonadal steroids (see Figure 1). The onset of puberty is heralded by a "decreased sensitivity" of the hypothalamic-pituitary axis to gonadal hormone feed-

FIGURE 1

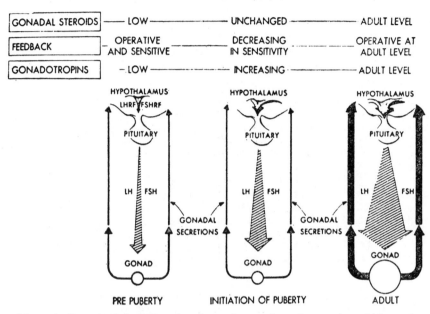

Schematic diagram of the progressive change in gonadotropin secretion which results from a decrease in hypothalamic sensitivity to gonadal steroids. (Reprinted from Reiter and Root, 1975.)

back control resulting in the increased production of gonadotropin releasing factors from the hypothalamus. In response to this stimulation, the anterior pituitary secretes gradually increasing levels of gonadotropins (luteinizing hormone (LH) and follicle stimulating hormone (FSH)) which result in increased production of gonadal hormones. Adult levels of gonadotropic and gonadal hormones are attained gradually, with LH reaching the adult level first, followed by FSH and the gonadal hormones. Hormonal levels have been correlated with stages of secondary sexual development.

The Adolescent Growth Spurt

The vast majority of increase in height for both sexes occurs during a span of 24 to 36 months and is termed the adolescent growth spurt. This spurt is characterized by an acceleration of linear growth velocity, a peak period of growth, which then is followed by a sharp

FIGURE 2

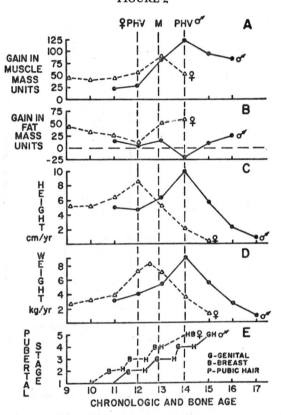

The mean changes in muscle mass, fat mass, height and weight as correlated to stage of pubertal development and mean chronologic age in normal males and females. PHV—peak height velocity. M—menarche. (Derived from Cheek, 1974; Marshall and Tanner, 1969, 1970; Tanner, 1962 and reproduced by permission of the authors and publishers.)

decline in growth velocity. Growth occurs in the same fashion for both sexes but its onset averages two years earlier and slightly less in magnitude in females (Barnes, 1975; Tanner, 1962). The onset of this growth spurt occurs in females between 9.5 years and 14.5 years; in males the onset can be between 10.5 years and 16 years (Figure 2C). In females the average age of peak growth is 12.1 years, with a peak velocity of 3.25 inches per year. Ninety-nine percent of growth has occurred by age 18 (Barnes, 1975).

In addition to linear growth, there are major changes in both the distribution and composition of body tissues. Both sexes have similar body composition and strength prior to puberty. With the onset of the growth spurt, the rate of fat accumulation decreases significantly for females, whereas males actually show an absolute loss of fat (Figure 2B). After peak growth has occurred, adipose tissue in females is rapidly added. Males add fat tissue more slowly and less quantitatively. The greater proportion of adipose tissue is decisive in the menstrual activity of the female. Approximately 17% body mass as fat is necessary for the onset of menstrual periods. Twenty-two percent body mass as fat is needed for continuation of regular ovulatory cycles (Frisch and McArthur, 1974).

The accumulation of muscle tissue, reflected as lean body mass, is significantly greater in the male than in the female (Figure 2A) after critical heights (different for each sex) have been achieved (Frisch and Revelle, 1971). Studies have shown that males not only have more muscle mass but also increased size of individual cells (Daniel, 1970). The distribution of muscle mass is significantly different in males and females, with males having greater concentration of muscle in the thighs, shoulders and back. These differences may be in response to the trophic effects of androgens, although this is far from conclusive (Daniel, 1970).

On the average, the adolescent doubles his ideal body weight during puberty. The manner in which weight is added is similar to that by which linear growth is attained (Figure 2D). There is an acceleration in velocity of weight gain, with a peak period of weight gain, followed by a decline in the velocity of weight gain. The curves reflecting weight gain are similar to those showing linear growth (Barnes, 1975).

The peak period of weight gain for the female occurs six months after her period of most rapid linear growth. In the male, however, the periods of peak linear growth and weight gain coincide. Thus, in contrast to linear growth, where the female peaks a full two years before the male, the female's peak weight gain occurs only an average of 18 months before that of the male.

With respect to changes in both weight and height, the velocity of change may vary. However, for each individual, the patterns of growth should be consistent so that, when weights and heights are plotted as a function of age, a smooth curve is obtained. Standard graphs plotting height versus age and weight versus age are readily available and can serve as accurate assessments of the progress of puberty. For any individual, normal growth should occur along a particular percentile without significant variation—assuming that percentile is not below the 3rd percentile nor above the 97th percentile, representing the lower and upper limits of normal, that is, ± 2 S.D. from the mean (Barnes, 1975; Kogut, 1973).

Secondary Sexual Characteristics

The hallmark of adolescence which most dramatically defines this period of life is the development of secondary sexual characteristics. Intimately related to these profound physical changes is much of the emotional turmoil that so characteristically engulfs the ever-changing adolescent. During this period of rapid bodily changes, the adolescent is constantly comparing himself to his peers. The professional who is actively involved with adolescents and who is at all sensitive realizes this intuitively. Understanding these changes and recognizing the various stages of maturity are important to the health care worker.

Secondary sexual development in the female begins with the development of breast buds (in 79%) or the growth of pubic hair (in 21%). According to Tanner's data, the mean ages for both are 11.2 years and 11.7 years, respectively (Marshall and Tanner, 1969). Despite these close means, however, it is important to realize that the correlation between breast development and pubic hair growth is variable. The initial onset of each, as well as the rapidity with which each stage is reached, is also variable (Marshall and Tanner, 1969).

Despite these variations in development, several definitive statements can be made. Using the mean ages for breast bud and pubic hair growth given above and defining normalcy as ±2 S.D. (i.e., 2.2 years and 2.4 years, respectively), then it follows that patients with breast development before 9 years should be assessed for premature thelarche if no pubic hair is present (Silver and Sami, 1968). Those with pubic hair growth before 9.3 years should be evaluated for premature pubarche (Barnes, 1975; Silverman et al., 1952). Conversely, assessment for delayed puberty should be considered if breast

TABLE 1

Stages of Secondary Sexual Development (Female)

Classification of sex maturity stages in girls

Stage	Pubic hair	Breasts
1	Preadolescent	Preadolescent
2	Sparse, lightly pigmented, straight, medial border of labia	Breast and papilla elevated as small mound; areolar diameter increased
3	Darker, beginning to curl, increased amount	Breast and areola enlarged, no contour separation
4	Coarse, curly, abundant but amount less than in adult	Areola and papilla form secondary mound
5	Adult feminine triangle, spread to medial surface of thighs	Mature; nipple projects, areola part of general breast contour

From Daniel, W. A., 1970.

development is delayed beyond 13.4 years or if the growth of pubic hair does not occur before 14.1 years (Barnes, 1975; Marshall and Tanner, 1969; Reiter and Kulin, 1972). Other extensive correlations between the various stages of breast and pubic hair growth have been made by Barnes (1975).

The various stages in the pubertal development of secondary sexual characteristics for females are described in Table 1. Menarche most commonly begins when most (60%) of females are at a stage of B-4 breast development (see Table 1) (Marshall and Tanner, 1969), which coincides to mean chronical age of 12.7 years. Ninety-nine percent of females will have onset of menarche within five years of breast budding. As already mentioned, the onset of menses is closely correlated with the percent of body fat.

Menstrual cycles are commonly irregular for the first several months and then often become relatively predictable. According to Zacharis, Wurtman and Schatzoff (1970), the mean age for onset of regular menses is 13.8 ±2 years. Thus, in the absence of associated symptoms, patients with irregular menstrual periods of less than two years' duration should be reassured. Those with irregular menses for longer than two years should have a full gynecological assessment (Barnes, 1975).

TABLE 2

Stages of Secondary Sexual Development (Male)

Classification of genitalia maturity stages in boys

Stage	Pubic hair	Penis	Testes
1	None	Preadolescent	
2	Slight, long, slightly pigmented	Slight enlargement	Enlarged scrotum, pink, texture altered
3	Darker, starts to curl, small amount	Penis longer	Larger
4	Resembles adult type, but less in quantity, coarse, curly	Larger, glans and breadth increase in size	Larger, scrotum dark
5	Adult distribution spread to medial surface of thighs	Adult	Adult

From Daniel, W. A., 1970.

Menarche before 10.3 years (12.7 ±2 S.D.) should be considered premature and should be evaluated. Conversely, the patient who has not had the onset of menses by age 15.5, assuming other parameters of growth and sexual maturation are normal, should be evaluated for primary amenorrhea.

The development of secondary sexual changes in the male follows comparable sequential stages descriptively outlined by Tanner and presented in Table 2. Male pubertal development is initiated by scrotal and testicular enlargement, with a mean age of onset being 11.6 years (Marshall and Tanner, 1969). Using 2 S.D. as the criteria for statistical normalcy, it follows that those males with onset before 9.5 years or after 13.6 years should be evaluated for precocious puberty and delayed puberty, respectively (Barnes, 1975; Marshall and Tanner, 1970; Stolz and Stolz, 1951).

As in female development, male genital and pubic hair development occur sequentially. However, the correlations between them vary, as do both the time of onset and the speed with which each stage is attained. Each should thus be staged separately (Barnes, 1975; Marshall and Tanner, 1970) . The average time between onset of scrotal/testicular enlargement and completion of genital development is 3.3 years (mean age 14.9 + 1.1 S.D.) (Marshall and Tanner, 1970) .

Although there is a great deal of individual variation, generally, axillary hair appears approximately two years after pubic hair growth begins; facial hair begins later and gradually reaches adult distribution (Barnes, 1975; Marshall and Tanner, 1970).

Stimulation of male breast development may occur in almost 30% of normal adolescents. Eighty percent will have nontender, bilateral gynecomastia, while about 20% of these males may have unilateral and/or tender breast masses (Barnes, 1975). Reassuring the adolescent male that he is normal may help greatly in alleviating anxiety associated with such development. The gynecomastia, which can develop rapidly over a period of several months, may require two years or more for resolution. It is suggested that breast tissue that is persistent beyond 18 months after its appearance or which severely disturbs the adolescent male should be surgically removed. Rarely is adolescent gynecomastia pathological (Barnes, 1975; Gallagher, Heald, and Garrell, 1976; Wilkins, 1948).

Figure 3 and Figure 4 present an overview of normal developmental variability and a comparison of onset and course of secondary

FIGURE 3

Female Secondary Sexual Development

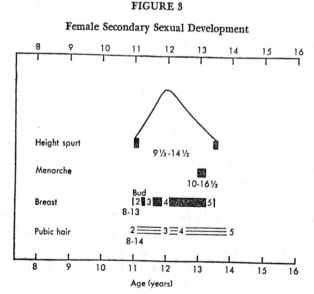

Variability of biologic maturity in girls. (From Tanner, J. M.: Growth at adolescence, ed. 2, Oxford, Engl., 1962, Blackwell Scientific Publications.)

FIGURE 4

Male Secondary Sexual Development

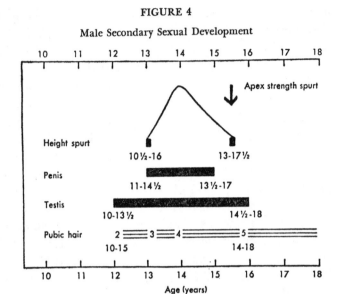

Variability of biologic maturity in boys. (From Tanner, J. M.: Growth at adolescence, ed. 2, Oxford, Engl., 1962, Blackwell Scientific Publications.)

sexual development between females (Figure 3) and males (Figure 4). Various "stages" refer to the well-known system of classification developed by Tanner. The adolescent psychiatrist, particularly, should be familiar with this important information.

Clinical Laboratory Results

A number of parameters can be correlated with the Tanner stages of secondary sexual development (see Tables 1 and 2). For example, serum alkaline phosphatase levels, which reflect bone osteoblastic activity, vary during puberty with peak mean values occurring at "sexual maturity stage two" in girls and at "stage three" in boys (see Figure 5). These values correlate well with peak height velocity changes in both sexes (Daniel, 1977).

Hematocrit values should be correlated with sex, race, and sexual maturity (Daniel, 1977). Variations with maturity rating are more noticeable for males than females (see Figure 6). These changes in males are related to increasing serum levels of testosterone, which stimulate the bone marrow directly as well as indirectly by requiring increased metabolic input for muscular growth and development.

FIGURE 5

Alkaline Phosphatase Levels

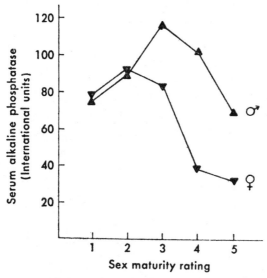

Relationship of serum alkaline phosphatase to SMR. (From Bennett, D. L., Ward, M. S., and
Daniel, Jr., W. A.: J. Pediatr. **88**:633, 1976.)

MEDICAL DISORDERS OF ADOLESCENCE

Medical disorders characteristic both of children and of adults can occur during adolescence. Therefore, the physician must keep in mind that he is dealing with a child-adult complex from a medical standpoint. Non-physician health care workers should also be attuned to certain disorders that might occur in which early diagnosis and treatment is important. Most of these disorders are endocrine in nature, while some, such as obesity and hypertension, have only indirect endocrinological manifestations.

It is always important to be aware of any medical problems that patients may be developing. However, most of these do not require a high index of suspicion to recognize a potential disorder. For example, if an adolescent complains of a sore throat, an earache, stomach cramps, burning on urination, or vaginal discharge, one knows he or she should see a physician. Some developing disorders

FIGURE 6

Hernatocrit Values

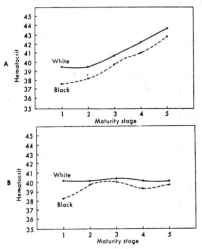

Hematocrit values for boys, A, and for girls, B. (From Daniel, W. A., Jr.: Pediatrics 52 |3|:388-394, 1973.)

may not be as apparent in the adolescent and can go undetected until much later. Early recognition of potential problems which may have lasting medical or psychosocial morbidity is a must in delivering total health care to the adolescent patient.

Therefore, this section deals with those medical disorders of adolescents which require a high index of suspicion to arrive at the diagnosis. These disorders are: 1) disorders of growth; 2) thyroid disease; 3) hypoglycemic states; 4) hypertensive states; and 5) chronic disease states. Obviously, conditions such as cancer, anemia, liver disease, breast masses, gastrointestinal disease or dysfunctional uterine bleeding can be associated with significant mortality or morbidity, but again most of these do not usually go undetected, because some sign or symptom brings the adolescent, with or without his parents, to the doctor. The conditions to be discussed here may go undetected because the adolescent and/or his parents are not aware of potential problems or the adolescent is too afraid or embarrassed to mention the problem.

Disorders of Growth

Disorders of growth constitute one of the main concerns of most adolescents. This concern may or may not be conveyed to the doctor. "I am too short, too tall, too fat or too thin" is a common complaint loudly—or not so loudly—voiced. Understanding the endocrinological aspects of puberty may be very reassuring to the patient and her doctor. For example, the four feet, eleven inch female who is only Tanner Stage 2 in breast and pubic hair may be concerned about not being five feet tall. The physician can examine her, plot her on a growth chart and, if all is well, reassure her that her development is progressing within normal limits. If the growth pattern is not that obvious, then a diagnostic approach is required. This approach requires a complete history, physical examination, certain laboratory and x-ray procedures and counseling.

Short stature is a concern at some point in time for most adolescents, especially males. It is the most common presenting complaint in most adolescent endocrine clinics. Since only 25% of adult males are six feet tall, the concern about stature is inevitable (American Academy of Pediatrics Committee on Drugs, 1977). The history and physical examination are basic to an evaluation of short stature. Most important in the history are the heights of family members for the previous two generations and the patient's past growth pattern. Gestational and perinatal history are also valuable indicators of antecedent events. Size at birth is not a good predictor, except possibly for premature infants.

On physical examination a head to toe, unclothed examination is a must. Height must be obtained with the patient standing without shoes and with heels, buttocks, shoulders and head touching the wall or measuring device. A growth chart to plot present height and weight values and to compare them to past values is important. The physician may then require a complete blood count, bone age film and special endocrine studies, depending on his assessment. After the work-up is completed counseling is necessary to deal with the feelings of the patient.

The differential diagnosis of those individuals two standard deviations below the mean is extensive. However, the main considerations are as follows: If the adolescent is short and obese, there is greater chance for an endocrine problem. The major disorders to be considered are: a) Cushings syndrome, b) hypothyroidism, c) Prader-Willi syndrome, d) Laurence-Moon Biedl syndrome, and e) gonadal dysgenesis syndromes. The other conditions to be considered are: a) familial short stature, b) constitutional short stature (i.e., delayed growth with retarded bone age and low serum alkaline phosphatase values), c) intrauterine growth retardation, d) emotional deprivation syndrome, e) hypopituitarism, f) dwarfism, g) inborn errors of metabolism, h) malabsorption syndromes, and i) chronic diseases, such as chronic renal failure of various etiologies.

The evaluation of tall stature is usually not as serious from a medical standpoint because it is not associated with underlying damaging pathology. However, it usually requires more counseling time, particularly with girls. The work-up should proceed as with short stature. Tallness in girls may not be socially desirable, whereas in males it is a desirable trait. If a girl is less than 11 years of age, has a skeletal age less than 11 years and has a predicted adult height of 5 feet 11 inches, prevention of this extent of growth should be considered (Daniel, 1977). If the decision is made by the parents and physician to use high-dose estrogen with cyclical progesterone and other hormonal therapy to prevent growth, an endocrinologist should follow the patient with a primary care physician.

The differential diagnosis of tall stature must include consideration of 1) genetic predisposition, 2) Marfan's syndrome, 3) pituitary tumors, and 4) chromosomal anomalies.

Obesity

Obesity is a disorder of growth that can be considered as a silent killer. Even when not so profound, it usually has major effects on the adolescent's physical and emotional health. All severe forms of obesity are the result of an excessive number of adipose cells. Hypercellular obesity begins in early childhood when it is felt there are critical periods during which the body's composition can be nutritionally programmed. Thus, for most adolescents, the pattern of obesity is already set and must be dealt with by behavior modification, often including the entire family. Obesity can be diagnosed if body weight is 20% or more above the ideal weight for height (Daniel, 1977).

Although most adolescent obesity is primarily exogenous in type, consideration must be given to several disorders that can have psychiatric components. Endocrine diseases such as hypothyroidism (especially in females), Cushing's syndrome or Stein-Leventhal syndrome, genetic diseases like Prader-Willi syndrome, and hypothalamic injury secondary to tumors or infection must initially be ruled out. Other rarer causes of obesity in adolescents must be considered in individual cases.

Anorexia Nervosa

The disorder of growth associated with being too thin that causes psychiatrists most concern is anorexia nervosa. If weight is greater than 15% below that appropriate for the individual's height, an evaluation for possible occult, chronic disease should be undertaken. Diseases such as chronic pyelonephritis, malabsorption secondary to various enzymatic and parasitic causes, cancer, endocrine disorders such as hyperthyroidism, and chronic recurrent bacterial and mycotic infections (especially pulmonary) should be excluded by appropriate testing.

If occult diseases are excluded and the following criteria are present, one should be concerned about impending anorexia: 1) a weight loss of at least 25% of original body weight, 2) amenorrhea, 3) a history of previous obesity, 4) negativism towards food, 5) a distorted body image, 6) periods of hyperactivity, and 7) an emotional conflict. Early recognition of this syndrome is a must so that appropriate behavioral and psychiatric intervention can occur.

Thyroid Disease

Thyroid diseases represent a considerable portion of the endocrine problems seen in adolescents, especially in females. Although most of the diseases seen are associated with noticeable enlargement of the thyroid, behavioral components such as emotional lability or depression (reflected in poor school performance or excessive fatigue) may precede noticeable physical changes by months. It may be difficult at times to differentiate these behaviors from the frequent, excessive mood swings normally present in adolescents.

The most common presentation of hyperthyroidism in adolescence is thyrotoxicosis (Graves' disease). Behavioral manifestations may commonly precede the physical stigmata (exopthalmos, enlarged thyroid, weight loss, and heat intolerance) and may occur suddenly or insidiously. Once the diagnosis is confirmed, appropriate medical management is usually possible, although a significant number of patients with Graves' disease may require subtotal resection with the concomitant risks of hypothyroidism and/or hypoparathyroidism.

Hypothyroidism may be enzymatic or autoimmune (Hashimoto's thyroiditis) in origin. Early recognition, diagnosis and management are crucial, since the ramifications of hypothyroidism in the adolescent can include delayed onset of puberty, subnormal growth, and retarded secondary sexual development. In the adolescent, these problems can have important secondary effects, distorting the adolescent's feelings of body image, self-esteem, and peer group relations.

Adolescent goiter, which can have multiple causes, usually presents itself as an enlarged neck mass with associated symptoms (depending upon the underlying cause). Thyroid carcinoma, which is very rare in adolescents unless neck irradiation has previously occurred, usually presents as a firm hard nodule with no associated cervical adenopathy. Thyroid scanning almost always shows decreased uptake whereas thyroid function tests are usually normal.

The impact of thyroid disease can be crucial to the adolescent's adjustment during the teenage years. Generally, hypothyroid patients respond better to therapy than do patients with hyperthyroidism.

Hypoglycemia

Hypoglycemia can present as a psychiatric disorder in the adolescent patient. Symptoms such as confusion, inability to concentrate, feelings of detachment from the environment, ataxia, dysarthria, visual disturbances, seizures or coma can be encountered, along with symptoms of catecholamine response such as flushing, sweating tremor, pallor or tachycardia. Conversely, it is possible (though more rare) to observe fatigue, depression or neurosis as the predominant manifestations of hypoglycemia.

A majority of patients experience post-prandial symptoms (stimulative hypoglycemia), whereas others complain of symptoms as late as eight hours after eating (fasting hypoglycemia). Diseases which produce fasting hypoglycemia are more likely to be serious. One must consider the following in the differential diagnosis of hypoglycemia: a) glycogen storage diseases, b) ketotic hypoglycemia, c) endocrine disorders, such as hypothyroidism, adrenal insufficiency, early diabetes or panhypopituitarism, d) hepatitis, e) pancreatic diseases such as beta cell hyperplasia, nesioblastosis, islet cell adenomas or Beckwith-Wiedemann Syndrome, f) extra pancreatic tumors, such as neuroblastoma, Wilms' Tumor, hepatoma or fibrosarcoma, g) malabsorption, h) poisons, and i) drugs such as insulin, alcohol, propranolol, and salicylates. By far the most common cause of hypoglycemia is diabetic insulin overdosage.

Hypertension

Hypertension is another medical disorder that may go unrecognized in the adolescent years. Its reported incidence has increased as blood pressure measurement has been routinely applied to adolescent health care. The acceptable upper limits of normal blood pressure in adolescents have not yet been standardized. It is probable that standards will more likely be correlated with parameters of growth and secondary sexual changes than with chronological age. Two questions must be answered when hypertension is recognized: 1) Is it persistent or transient? 2) Is it essential or secondary to another disease? The presenting signs and symptoms will help answer these two questions.

All acutely ill patients, especially those with involvement of the central nervous, cardiovascular or renal systems, should have their blood pressure measured. The differential diagnosis is extensive, although essential hypertension may account for between 30% and 50% of all cases seen. Renal, cardiovascular, endocrine and drug-related (especially stimulants, oral contraceptives, LSD, PCP) causes must be considered.

Chronic Illness

Chronic diseases occur in adolescents with a higher frequency than is commonly recognized. Mattsson (1972) defined a chronic illness as "a disorder with a protracted course which can be progressive and fatal, or associated with a relatively normal life span despite impaired physical and mental functioning." Diseases like ulcerative colitis, Crohn's disease, cystic fibrosis, diabetes mellitus, chronic renal failure (of various causes), some types of heart disease, juvenile rheumatoid arthritis, scoliosis, and leukemia and other curable forms of cancer have secondary effects which can become more difficult to treat than the primary illness.

Adolescent responses may include social isolation and/or withdrawal from peers, regression, aggressive behavior, neurotic dependency, low self-esteem and depression. Parents and siblings may experience periods of crises marked by guilt, embarrassment, grief, resentment, chronic sorrow and acceptance. The particular responses result from the "nature of the illness itself, the attendant medical procedures, or the emotional reactions of the ill individual and family members to the illness" (Leichtman and Friedman, 1975).

In evaluation of the adolescent (and family) with a chronic disease, particular attention should be given to the timing of the disease's onset with respect to the adolescent's physical and psychosexual development. The achievement of the psychosocial tasks of adolescence may be inhibited, delayed, partially accomplished or normally completed depending on the interaction between the physical and emotional stresses of the adolescent period (cf. Battle, 1975; Leichtmann and Friedman, 1975; Mattsson, 1972).

CONCLUSION

A basic understanding of the endocrinology of puberty and of medical problems common to adolescence is of crucial importance to the adolescent psychiatrist. Non-medical therapists should also have some degree of awareness of these problems. A holistic view of the adolescent and an understanding of the impact of physiology and physical illness will make the mental health professional more effective in meeting the total health care needs of the adolescent patient.

REFERENCES

AMERICAN ACADEMY OF PEDIATRICS, COMMITTEE ON DRUGS. Counseling and synthetic steroids in short stature with organic disease. *Pediatrics,* 53:285-287, 1977.

BARNES, H. V. Physical growth and development during puberty. *Med. Clin. North America,* 59(6):1305, 1975.

BATTLE, C. U. Chronic physical disease. *Pediatric Clinic of North America,* 22:525, 1975.

BENNETT, D. L., WARD, M. S., & DANIEL, W. A., JR. Relationship of serum alkaline phosphatase contributions to sex maturity ratings in adolescents. *J. Pediatr.,* 88:633, 1976.

CHEEK, D. B. Body composition, hormones, nutrition and adolescent growth. In N. M. Grumbach, G. D. Grave, & F. E. Mayer (Eds.), *Control of Onset of Puberty.* New York: J. Wiley and Sons, 1974.

DANIEL, W. A. *The Adolescent Patient.* St. Louis, Mo.: C. V. Mosby, 1970.

DANIEL, W. A., JR. Hematocrit: Relationship to adolescence. *Pediatrics,* 5 (3):388-394, 1973.

DANIEL, W. A. *Adolescents in Health and Disease.* St. Louis, Mo.: C. V. Mosby, 1977.

FRISCH, R. E. & MCARTHUR, J. W. Menstrual cycles: Fatness as a determinant of minimum weight for height necessary for their maintenance or onset. *Science,* 185:949, 1974.

FRISCH, R. E. & REVELLE, R. The height and weight of girls and boys at the time of initiation of the adolescent growth spurt and the relationship to menarche. *Human Biol.,* 43:140-159, 1971.

GALLAGHER, J. R., HEALD, F. P., & GARELL, D. C. *Medical Care of the Adolescent* (3rd edition). New York: Appleton-Century-Crofts. 1976.

KOGUT, M. D. Growth and development in adolescence. *Pediatr. Clin. North America,* 20(4):789, 1973.

LEICHTMANN, S. R. & FRIEDMAN, S. B. Social and psychological development of adolescents and the relationship to chronic illness. *Med. Clin. North America,* 59 (6): 1319, 1975.

MARSHALL, W. A. & TANNER, J. M. Variations in patterns of pubertal changes in girls. *Arch. Dis. Child.,* 44:291, 1969.

MARSHALL, W. A. & TANNER, J. M. Variations in patterns of pubertal changes in boys. *Arch. Dis. Child.,* 45:13, 1970.

MATTSSON, A. Long-term physical illness in childhood: A challenge to psychosocial adaptation. *Pediatrics,* 50:801-811, 1972.

REITER, E. O. & KULIN, H. E. Sexual maturation in the female. *Ped. Clin. No. America,* 19(3):581, 1972.

REITER, E. O. & ROOT, A. W. Hormonal changes of adolescence. *Med. Clin. N. Amer.,* 59(6):1289, 1975.

SILVER, H. D. & SAMI, D. Premature thelarche: Precocious development of the breast. *Pediatrics,* 34:107, 1968.

SILVERMAN, S. H., ET AL. Precocious growth of sexual hair without other secondary sexual development: Premature pubarche a constitutional variation of adolescence. *Pediatrics,* 10:426, 1952.

STOLZ, H. R. & STOLZ, L. M. *Somatic Development of Adolescent Boys.* New York: Macmillan, 1951.

TANNER, J. M. *Growth at Adolescence,* 2nd Ed. Oxford, England: Blackwell Scientific Publications, 1962.

WILKINS, L. Abnormalities and variations in sexual development during childhood and adolescence. *Adv. Pediatr.,* 3:159, 1948.

ZACHARIS, L., WURTMAN, R. J., & SCHATZOFF, M.: Sexual maturation in contemporary American girls. *Am. J. Obstet. Gynecol.,* 108:833, 1970.

4

Normal Adolescent Development

DANIEL OFFER, M.D.

Why has the empirical study of normality and health been a relative newcomer in adolescent psychiatry and in all behavioral science investigations? One obvious reason is that it is a result of training, in that training procedures not only are a set of skills but are what Kaplan (1967) calls a "trained incapacity." Trained to recognize the abnormal, the adolescent psychiatrist and other behavioral scientists have had difficulty with recognizing, let alone conceptualizing, the normal. Yet, it is important to study normality because it serves as a baseline for all behavior.

WHAT DO WE MEAN BY NORMAL?

A review of social and behavioral science literature on normality led to a categorization of views on normality as belonging within four functional perspectives (Offer and Sabshin, 1974). Although each perspective is unique and has its own definition and description, the perspectives do complement each other and together they represent the total behavioral and social science approach to normality. Brief descriptions of the four perspectives follow.

The first perspective, *normality as health,* is basically the traditional medical psychiatric approach to health and illness. Most physicians equate normality with health and view health as an almost universal phenomenon. As a result, behavior is assumed to be within normal limits when no manifest psychopathology is present. If doctors were to transpose all behavior upon a scale, normality would encompass the major portion of the continuum and abnormality would be the small remainder. This definition of normality correlates with the traditional role model of the doctor who attempts to free his patient from grossly observable signs and symptoms. To this physician, the lack of pathological signs or symptoms indicates health. In other words, health in this context refers to a *reasonable* rather than an *optimal* state of functioning. In its simplest form, this perspective is illustrated by Romano (1950), who stated that a healthy person is one who is reasonably free of undue pain, discomfort, and disability.

The second perspective, *normality as utopia,* conceives of normality as that harmonious and optimal blending of the diverse elements of the mental apparatus that culminates in optimal functioning. Such a definition emerges clearly when psychiatrists or psychoanalysts talk about the ideal person or when they grapple with a complex problem such as discussing their criteria of successful treatment. This approach can be ascribed directly to Freud who, when discussing normality in 1937, stated: "A normal ego is like normality in general, an ideal fiction." While this approach is characteristic of a significant segment of psychoanalysts, it is by no means unique. It can also be found among psychotherapists in the field of psychiatry and psychology of quite different persuasions.

The third perspective, *normality as average,* is commonly employed in normative studies of behavior and is based on a mathematical principle of the bell-shaped curve. This approach conceives of the middle range as "normal" and *both* extremes as deviant. The normative approach, which is based on the statistical principle, describes each individual in terms of general assessment and total score. Variability is described only within the context of one individual. Although this approach is more commonly used in psychology and biology than in psychiatry, psychiatrists have been recently using pencil and paper tests to a much larger extent than in the past. Not only do psychiatrists utilize results of IQ tests, Rorschach, or Thematic Apperception Tests, but they also construct their own tests and questionnaires. In developing model personalities for different societies, one assumes that the typologies of character can be statistically measured.

The fourth perspective, *normality as transactional systems,* stresses that normal behavior is the end result of interacting systems. Based on this definition, temporal changes are essential to a complete definition of normality. In other words, the normality-as-transactional-systems perspective stresses changes or processes rather than a cross-sectional definition of normality. Investigators who subscribe to this approach can be found in all the behavioral and social sciences. Most typical is Grinker's (1956) thesis of a unified theory of behavior encompassing polarities within a wide range of integration. The interest in general system theory (von Bertalanffy, 1968) has further stressed the general applicability of the general system research for psychiatry. Normality as transactional systems encompasses variables from the biological, psychological, and social fields, all contributing to the functioning of a viable system over time. It is the integration of the variables into the system and the loading (or significance) assigned to each variable that will have to be more thoroughly explored in the future.

These four functional perspectives of normality can be applied both conceptually and empirically to any stage in the life cycle. By tracing a theory of personality development to its conceptual base, we will be better able to understand its place within the larger field. Since the goal in this chapter is to describe normal adolescent development, we will return to the four perspectives of normality whenever indicated in order to better understand the place of personal bias of the investigator (i.e. his chosen perspectives) in his theory or findings.

The field of adolescent development has never suffered from underexposure in the contemporary social and behavioral science scene. Whether in theory, therapy, psychopathology, problems and solutions, we have seen and read all there is to see and read. Much of the rest of this volume will address itself to many of these problems. It is therefore not necessary to dwell on it in this chapter. There have been only a handful of follow-up studies of normal adolescents. Some of these will be reviewed, particularly in the context of describing my own study of normal adolescent boys in detail. We will make a few comments on the developmental psychology of girls as well, although the empirical data on which our comments will be based are meager at best. During the past two decades there have been seven times more studies on adolescent boys than adolescent girls. We hope that the new generation of investigators will take this into account. We are trying to do our share and have just begun a longitudinal study of adolescent girls (Petersen, Offer, and Solomon, 1979).

Research on normal populations is not exclusively of recent origin. Anthropologists have been observing cultures other than their own for ever 70 years. Social psychologists and child psychologists have worked with normal people in experimental and testing situations ever since psychology began functioning as a scientific discipline. Psychoanalysts, although studying only patients who come to see them for psychoanalysis or psychotherapy, have extended their theories to include concepts applicable to the personality development of normal children and adults. What has been lacking, in our opinion, are systematic studies via longitudinal or follow-up studies of normal populations. We need to integrate the clinicians' experience and abilities with the researcher's tools and methods (Offer, Freedman and Offer, 1972).

In reviewing the findings from the more important psychiatric and clinical studies on normal populations which have been undertaken during the past decade, let us begin with a historical note. The two most influential and pioneering works on the psychology of normal populations were Grinker and Spiegel's *Men Under Stress* (1945) and White's *Lives in Progress* (1952). Both works describe coping mechanisms of nonpatient, or normal, populations. Grinker and Spiegel studied the behavior and psychological functioning of soldiers under combat conditions. White, via interviews, followed the lives of a selected group of college students. He assessed their success or failure in adaptation to their internal and external environment and their overall psychological competence. Both pioneering works fell short on methodology, but they laid the groundwork for the more solid empirical work which followed.

Rather than review the literature on normal adolescent development, we wish to concentrate on the findings which stem from the few longitudinal studies on adolescent development. It seems to us that the following studies are the ones which have dealt with the problem of how normal adolescents develop and the kind of psychological problems with which they have to cope during the adolescent process: Symonds and Jensen, 1961; Cox, 1970; Vaillant, 1977; King, 1971; Block, 1971; Grinker and Werble, 1974; Offer, 1973; and Offer & Offer, 1975. These longitudinal studies, although they vary in methodology and in the span of years they cover, have come up with remarkably similar results. All of them deal only with white middle-class adolescents.

In the remainder of this chapter we will describe in detail the findings which stem from our study of normal adolescent males. This study is an empirical one which does not claim to have discovered the only typology of normal adolescent development. It does, however, describe how one group of normal adolescent males progresses through the adolescent years. Our theories concerning adolescent development have to encompass this group as well as any other.

THE MODAL ADOLESCENT STUDY

This is a study of middle-class, Midwestern adolescent males. They went to high school in suburban communities, and most of them went on to college. The subjects saw us first when they were 14, and last when they were 22. We began in 1962 and studied 73 subjects throughout high school and 61 for four more years. The access to information about them during their high school years, as well as for four years afterwards, provided a longitudinal perspective giving us a view of how they have or have not changed while their environments changed. The sample included a few black and Latin American adolescents. The percentage of minority group adolescents in our sample (7%) was the same as the percentage of the minority group populations in the suburbs studied. However, the number is too small to enable us to draw meaningful conclusions regarding the developmental psychology of minority group adolescents.

The Selection Process

The *normality as average* perspective was utilized for selecting the study population. Two suburban high schools were chosen whose population represented the full range of the middle class.

A Self-Image Questionnaire was constructed. It was administered to students in the two entering freshman classes. The Self-Image Questionnaire was designed to evaluate the adolescent functioning in multiple areas. Students whose answers fell within one standard deviation from the mean in at least nine out of ten scales were selected as subjects for our study. The aim was to find a modal population and to eliminate the extremes of psychopathology, deviancy, and superior adjustment. There were no volunteers—we wanted to do the selection.

Information concerning the subjects was solicited from teachers and parents in order to further insure that the deviants within the group were not included. In the three cases where there was strong disagreement between the teachers' ratings and the test data, the subjects were not included in the study. The parents of the subjects selected were also asked to inform the researchers whether their children had had psychiatric treatment or whether for any reason the parents believed that their children were maladjusted. No parent gave any reason to reject their child on these grounds, though a couple expressed surprise that their children were called "normal."

The SIQ data which were used for selecting the normal subjects, preliminary to the more thorough investigation, can now be placed within a larger population context. The Questionnaire has been administered to over 20,000 teenagers. The samples include males and females, psychiatric patients, nonpatients, delinquents, younger and older adolescents (urban and suburban) in 40 different metropolitan centers in the United States, Australia, Ireland, Israel, Mexico, India, and Brazil. Cross-cultural differences have emerged.

The results have supported the contention that the test taps significant areas in the life of adolescents (Offer, Ostrov and Howard, 1977). Responses of emotionally disturbed teenagers have differed significantly from responses of delinquent and nonpatient normal populations. Males were different from females; younger teenagers were different from older teenagers. The belief that our original selection was, in fact, a selection from two relatively non-pathological high school populations has been confirmed. The subjects were within the mainstream of a middle-class, 13-to14-year-old, nonpatient, male youth. Other populations (e.g., rural and inner-city teenagers) have been tested from 1962 to the present. No subgroupings by time have emerged. For psychodynamic purposes, age and sex of the adolescent have had more of a differentiating effect than the year in which the test was administered. (See, for example, Welsh & Offer, 1978.)

THE LONGITUDINAL STUDY: NORMALITY AS
TRANSACTIONAL SYSTEMS

Once the subjects had been selected, the perspective on normality shifted. Normality as average was no longer to be the major mode of evaluating this group. For a further in-depth personality study one need not rely on the kind of behavioral data that often must be utilized in numerically larger studies. We had the facilities, the time, and the cooperation of the subjects so that we could now concentrate more on differing patterns of meaning for each individual's set of responses. The *normality as transactional systems* approach was utilized for describing the population that was being studied. Within this approach changes or processes are the crucial variants of normality; cross-sectional static definitions of normality are useful only as they play a role within the broader field approach.

The Data Collection

The main instrument for the collection of data was the semi-structured psychiatric, or clinical, interview. Other procedures were utilized as well so that bias of the experimenter (or interviewer) expectancy (Rosenthal, 1966) would be minimized. Thus, in addition to the psychiatric interviews of the subjects and of their parents, teachers' ratings and psychological testing were undertaken. The sociologists who conducted the survey interviews and the psychologists who administered the psychological testing did not share their findings with the psychiatrists until their part of the project was completed. Thereby, we ensured that the different sources of data would be independently collected. Gathering data on the subjects through these different research techniques was done in order to increase the validity of the conclusions which would eventually be drawn from the data.

Initially, the project had been designed as a four-year study.

Subjects had been asked to take part in the research only while they were in high school. In the fall of 1966 we mailed a letter to the subjects' former home addresses asking for their cooperation in the post high school segment of the project.

The 61 subjects who were studied post high school selected the following activities during their first year after graduating from high school: college—45 subjects (74%); the Armed Forces—eight (13%); and work—eight (13%).

Ten subjects whose families had moved away from the Chicago area could not be located. Of those who were contacted, two refused to participate. Thus, follow-up data on 61 out of the original 73 subjects, or 84% of the original sample, were available. Fifty of the subjects have been interviewed and 39 have been given a repeat psychological testing.

Data Analysis

An examination of the clinical as well as the statistical groupings of the subjects participating in the modal adolescent project resulted in a differentiation of psychological growth patterns of normal adolescents. An analysis of the data using appropriate statistical techniques (factor and typal analysis) revealed that even within our group chosen for qualities of homogeneity there were three subgroupings of adolescents. These subgroupings made clinical as well as statistical sense.

After working with these subjects for a period of eight to ten years, we knew each one as an individual above and beyond his statistical scores on a variety of tests and measurements. By studying the clinical material on the subjects in each of the three subgroups, the psychological similarity of the subjects within each of the subgroups and their differences from members of the other subgroups could be identified. These similarities are apparent not only by referring to the factor scores, but also through subjective clinical impressions, which, of course, were one basis on which the factor scores were constructed.

A complex interaction of biopsychosocial variables, such as child-rearing practices, genetic background, experiential factors, cultural and social surroundings, and the psychological defenses and coping mechanisms of the individual, make up the growth patterns.

The three groups have been labeled by the growth patterns they have shown throughout the eight-year course of the study. The groups* are:

1. Continuous Growth Group	(23%)
2. Surgent Growth Group	(35%)
3. Tumultuous Growth Group	(21%)

CONTINUOUS GROWTH

The subjects described within the Continuous Growth grouping developed from adolescents to young men with a smoothness of purpose and a self-assurance of their progression toward a meaningful and fulfilling adult life. These subjects were favored by circumstances. Their genetic and environmental backgrounds were excellent. Their childhood had been unmarked by death or serious illnesses of a parent a sibling. The nuclear family remained a stable unit throughout their childhood and adolescence. The Continuous Growth subjects had mastered previous developmental stages without serious setbacks. These subjects accepted general cultural and societal norms and felt comfortable within them. They had a capacity to integrate experiences and use them as a stimulus for growth.

The parents were able to encourage their children's independence; they themselves grew and changed with their children. There was basic respect, trust, and affection between the generations. The ability to allow their sons' independence in many areas was undoubtedly facilitated by the sons' growth patterns. Since the young men were not behaving in a manner clearly divergent from that of the parents, the parents could continue to be provided with need-gratifications through their sons. The sons were gaining both from the parents' good feelings toward them and the parental willingness to allow them to create their own individual lives outside of the household. The value system of the subjects in this group dovetailed with that of the parents. In many ways, the young men were functioning as continuations of the parents, living out not so much lives the parents had wished for but not attained, but rather lives similar to those of the parents.

---

* (21% mixed scores; they were dropped for this analysis).

As regards their interpersonal relationships, the subjects had close male friends in whom they could confide or a group of friends with whom they shared experiences. Their relationships with the opposite sex became increasingly important as they reached the post high school years.

Subjects described by the Continuous Growth pattern acted in accordance with their consciences, manifesting little evidence of superego problems and developing meaningful ego ideals, often identifying with persons whom they knew and admired within the larger family unit, the school, the community, or the American political arena. These subjects were able to identify feelings of shame and guilt, and proceeded to explain not only how the experiences provoking these responses had affected them, but also how they brought closure to the uncomfortable situations (action orientation). A second similar experience might be described then by these young men, but one which they had been prepared to handle better, putting the earlier upsetting experience into a past time of immaturity conquered.

Although these young men could dream about being the best in the class, their actions were guided by a pragmatic and realistic appraisal of their own abilities and of external circumstances. Thus, they were prevented from meeting with repeated disappointments.

The subjects were able to cope with external trauma, usually through an adaptive action orientation. When difficulties arose, they used the defenses of denial and isolation to protect themselves from being bombarded with affect. They could postpone immediate gratification and work in a sustained manner for a future goal. Temporary suppression, rather than repression, of affect allowed them to modulate their aggressive and sexual impulses without being overwhelmed or acting out in a self-destructive manner. They did not experience prolonged periods of anxiety or depression—two of the most common affects described by the entire subject population, including this subgroup.

The qualities which were common to members of this group were many of those which appear when mental health is viewed in an ideal sense. The individuals of the Continuous Growth Group would, of course, never portray all of these qualities, but would have some difficulties in one or another area. What was most distinctive about members of the Continuous Growth Group was their overall contentment with themselves and their place in life. When compared to the other two groupings, this group was composed of relatively happy human beings. They generally had an order to their lives which could be interrupted but which did not yield to states of symptomatology or chaotic behavior as these young men progressed through the adolescent years and matured cognitively and emotionally.

None of the subjects in this group had received psychotherapy or was thought by the researchers to need treatment. This is not surprising since the person seeking psychotherapy as an adolescent or young adult would be unlikely to be characterized as belonging in the category of Continuous Growth. The significance of the finding that none of these subjects were seen by psychotherapists or counselors from the health services of the schools or communities lies in the fact that they are then least likely to be the young adults from whom members of the helping professions build their studies or make their generalizations about youth populations.

SURGENT GROWTH

The Surgent Growth Group, although functioning as adaptively as was the first group, was characterized by important enough differences to present a different cluster and to be defined as a different subgroup. Developmental spurts are illustrative of the pattern of growth of the Surgent Growth Group. These subjects differed in the amount of emotional conflicts. There was more concentrated energy directed toward mastering developmental tasks than was obvious for members of the Continuous Growth Group. At times these subjects would be adjusting very well, integrating their experiences and moving ahead, and at other times they seemed to be temporarily immobilized within certain developmental areas. A cycle of progression and regression is more typical of this group than of the Continuous Growth Group.

One of the major differences between the Surgent Growth subjects and those in the Continuous Growth Group was that their genetic and/or environmental backgrounds were not as free of problems and traumas; the nuclear families in the Surgent Growth Group were more likely to have been affected by separation, death, or severe illnesses.

Although subjects in this category were able to cope with their "average expectable environment" (Hartmann, 1958), unanticipated problems would inevitably arise. Affects which were usually flexible and available would, at the time of crisis, become stringently controlled. This, together with the fact that they were not as action-oriented as the first group, made them slightly more prone to depression. The depression would accompany or follow the highly controlled behavior. On other occasions, when their defense mechanisms faltered they experienced moderate anxiety, with a short period of turmoil resulting. There was a tendency to use projection and anger.

These subjects were not as confident as were the young men in the Continuous Growth Group; their self-esteem wavered. They relied more heavily upon positive reinforcement from the opinions of important others, such as parents and/or peers. As a group, they were able to form meaningful interpersonal relationships similar to those of individuals in the Continuous Growth Group. The relationships, though, were be maintained with a greater degree of effort.

For subjects described under the Surgent Growth category, relationships with parents were marked by conflicts of opinions and values. There were areas of disagreement between father and mother concerning basic issues such as the importance of discipline, academic attainments, or religious beliefs. The mothers of some of these subjects had more difficulty in letting their children grow and in separating from them.

The subjects might work toward their vocational goals sporadically or with a lack of enthusiasm, but they would be able to keep their long-range behavior in line with their general expectations for themselves.

There were subjects in this group who were afraid of emerging sexual feelings and impulses. For these young adults, meaningful relationships with the opposite sex began in the post high school years, except for a small subgroup who started experimenting with sexuality early in high school, possibly owing to needs for reassurance. These early sexual relationships were not lasting, although they could be helpful in overcoming anxiety concerning sexuality.

The group as a whole was less introspective than either the first or the third group. Overall adjustment of these subjects was often just as adaptive and successful as that of the first group. The adjustment was achieved, though, with less self-examination and a more controlled drive or surge toward development, with suppression of emotionality being characteristic of the subjects in the Surgent Growth Group.

TUMULTUOUS GROWTH

The third group, the Tumultuous Growth Group, is similar to the adolescents so often described in psychiatric, psychoanalytic, and social science literature. These are the students who go through adolescence with internal turmoil which manifests itself in overt behavioral problems in school and at home. These adolescents have been observed to have recurrent self-doubts, escalating conflicts with their parents and debilitating inhibitions. They often respond inconsistently to their social and academic environments.

Subjects characterized by a tumultuous growth pattern were those who experienced growing up from 14 to 22 as a period of discordance, as a transitional period for which their defenses needed mobilizing and adaptational abilities needed to be learned or reinforced.

The subjects demonstrating Tumultuous Growth patterns came from less stable backgrounds than did those subjects in the other two groups. More of the parents in this group had irreconcilable marital conflicts and others had a history of mental illness in the family. Also present was a social class difference. The study population was primarily middle-class but this group contained many subjects who belonged to the lower-middle-class. For them, functioning in a middle- and upper-middle-class environment (the two suburbs within which the study was conducted) might have been a cause for additional stresses.

The Tumultuous Growth Group experienced more events as major psychological trauma. The difficulties in their life situation were more evident than the satisfactions. Defenses were not well developed for handling emotionally trying situations. A relatively high percentage of this group had overt clinical problems and had received psychotherapy.

Separation was painful to the parents and became a source of continuing conflict for the subjects. The parent-son relationships characterizing this group were similar to those of many of the neurotic adolescents seen in outpatient psychotherapy. Further, parent-son communication of a system of values was poorly defined or contradictory.

Strong family bonds, however, were present within the Tumultuous Growth Group as they were within each of the growth patterns. We had one test for evaluating strength and openness of family communication, utilizing the revealed differences technique. This method clearly differentiated the families of our modal sample along the three developmental routes. Understanding between the generations was observed most often in the Continuous Growth Group and least often in the Tumultuous Growth Group, with the Surgent Group in between.

The ability of the Tumultuous Growth Group to test reality and act accordingly was relatively strong in contrast to patient populations, but disappointment in others and in themselves when contrasted to other nonpatient populations was prevalent. Changes in self-concept could precipitate moderately severe anxiety reactions. Mood swings accompanied their search for who they were as separate individuals and concern about whether their activities were worthwhile. Feelings of mistrust about the adult world were often expressed by subjects in this group.

Affect was readily available and created both intensely pleasurable and painful experiences. Action was accompanied by more anxiety and depression in this group than in the other two groups. Emotional turmoil was part of their separation-individuation process. Without the tumult, growth toward independence and meaningful interpersonal relationships was in doubt.

These subjects were considerably more dependent on peer culture than were their age-mates in the other groups, possibly because they received fewer gratifications from their relationships within the family. When they experienced a personal loss, such as the ending of a relationship with a good friend, their depression was deeper, though only very rarely associated with suicidal feelings and impulses.

The Tumultuous Growth subjects had begun dating activities at a younger age than their peers described in the first two groups.

For some, in early adolescence their relationships with females were characterized by dependency. In late adolescence, their heterosexual relationships generally gained added meaning, as they became able to appreciate the personal characteristics of their female friends.

Many subjects in the Tumultuous Growth Group were highly sensitive and introspective individuals. They were usually aware of their emotional needs. Academically, they were less interested in science, engineering, law and medicine, and preferred the arts, the humanities, or the social and psychological sciences. However, business and engineering careers remained the most usual choices for this group as well as for the first two groups.

As with other variables, academic success differentiated the groups, but honor students and average students or workers could be found within each group. The academic or work failures were more likely to be found in the Tumultuous Group, since they would find the tasks upon which they had embarked to be incompatible with their needs or abilities only after having tried them.

The adolescents in this grouping experienced more psychological pain than did the others; however, as a group, they were not, as a result, living less meaningful lives in terms of their overall functioning within their respective environmental settings than were the persons in the Continuous and Surgent Growth groups. They were less happy with themselves and more critical of their social environment, but could be just as successful academically or vocationally.

SUMMARY AND CONCLUSION

We have seen that, during the adolescent years, the adolescent completes many aspects of mature development and is still working on others. After high school, young people are physically mature and are most likely to have attained their peak cognitive development, though knowledge can, of course, continuously increase. Psychosocial development, on the other hand, has come a long way but is by no means complete. Forming an identity (sexual, vocational, moral, social) is the major psychosocial task of adolescence, but the development of some aspects of identity continues throughout life.

From the Eriksonian (1959) point of view, our subjects have achieved temporal perspective and, in fact, appear to have a heightened awareness of time. Self-certainty is a more difficult task to master; many individuals show some degree of self-consciousness throughout life. Egocentrism is less prevalant during post high school years than in high school.

Many youth in the post high school years are still actively experimenting with roles. For others, role fixation is a realistic limitation on future opportunities. Most youth are beginning, at least, to seriously consider occupational choices. Most have begun to develop intimate interpersonal and sexual relationships.

The last two conflicts of the adolescent crisis—leadership and followership versus authority confusion, and ideological commitment versus confusion of values—will probably not be resolved even in college. Most college-age youths are actively struggling with these issues with relatively few actually resolving them much before the end of college.

Our study demonstrates that about one-fourth of the modal sample progressed continuously and developed values similar to those of their parents. A second group developed by spurts with periodic turmoil. The third group experienced the years from 14 to 22 with the turmoil frequently generalized to all adolescents. For them, the development tasks leading to an identity were difficult.

There is good evidence that parents are especially important to adolescent development. Well-adjusted parents can facilitate development in this period, while conflicted parents may exacerbate difficulties. This finding about parents is equally applicable to our society. History suggests that adolescents have greater difficulty making the transition to adulthood when the society itself is in turmoil. It is important to recognize which manifestations are related to adolescence and which are more specific to a particular society at a particular point in time.

By the end of high school most youth are capable of living independently from their families and making their own decisions. We may question their judgment but, as adults, they must begin to experience their own successes and failures. The turmoil of adolescence, if it occurred, has now subsided—not into calm but into a more controlled, reasoned approach to the many problems presented by life.

Our longitudinal study (Offer and Offer, 1975) points to continuity between generations and continuity of coping styles throughout one's life. From 14 to 22, changes in appearance and changes in ability to make judgments were prevalent far more than were changes in levels of functioning, changes in defenses, or changes in one's emotional equilibrium.

Studies which differentiate developmentally between groups of adolescents should help us to identify the various healthy coping mechanisms and learn to what extent they, as well as age-specific tasks, characterize adolescence as a stage apart. Then we can look at the patient who needs help with a less limited conceptualization of the possibilities of adolescent development. Or, if the patient belongs in the category of tumultuous development, we will be able to isolate his problems more specifically along his own developmental lines rather than along the necessities of his age.

What the three route divisions do show us is the fallacy in many of the generalizations made for the period of adolescence. When depicting a period of adolescence, to know primarily the generalizations is not more useful than to classify all patients in one diagnostic category. Thus we need to understand varieties within psychodynamic formulations of normal adolescence. Rather than characterizing adolescence only as a unique stage apart, we should understand it according to its more particular manifestations and as one transitional period which will probably be more true to individual character styles than to any stage-specific capsule formulations.

For the adolescent in general, we should know that his rebellion against society is not to be programmed into our plans for him. And if he does not change our world as he grows older, perhaps it is because he never really wanted to. Our assessment of the young and our goals for a better world to come should not lead to disappointment in the young who will not lead us there or to a crushing of their independence because we fear that they may be leading us astray. The fears and the hopes are probably theirs as well as ours, because so we have bred them.

FURTHER RESEARCH NEEDS

We are a long way yet from totally understanding this period of life. A major contribution to our understanding would be from studies taking a more integrated approach to this stage of life. Each discipline has its own theories and methodologies which tell us a great deal about particular aspects of the problem. But it is frequently difficult to integrate these results in a way that permits a comprehensive understanding of either the stage of life or any individual.

We have discussed adolescent development from the psychosocial point of view since our empirical data base was applicable to it. We did not touch the other two broad areas: the physiological and the cognitive. We lack systematic research which integrates development among these spheres. The existing theories of development do not integrate these aspects in a comprehensive way though psychoanalytic theory comes closest.

We find it particularly important to integrate clinical observations with developmental research. Only by understanding normal development can we understand its deviations. For example, by comparing factors involved in normal development with those in delinquency or psychopathology we may learn how problems develop and hence be better able to plan effective interventions. Similarly, the study of psychopathology or delinquency will point to problem areas and will greatly enhance our understanding of the significant aspects of normal development. For example, it would tell us a great deal about normal development to know why schizophrenia seldom appears earlier than adolescence. In addition, the study of treatment course also tells us a great deal about human development and its influences.

We therefore stress the importance of a systems theory approach to clinical research focusing on the relevant problems of adolescent development. Clinicians and researchers working together can greatly enhance their individual efforts.

Finally, as we noted at the beginning of this chapter, our understanding of normal adolescence is based primarily on white, middle-class males. Very few studies have included blacks or other minority groups. And while there have been more studies of females in the past few years, there still are very few on populations younger than college-age. Probably because most research is done with college populations, or in college communities, lower-class groups are seldom included. Studies with these populations of adolescents may greatly alter our understanding of this stage of life.

REFERENCES

BLOCK, J. *Lives Through Time.* Berkeley: Bancroft, 1971.

COX, R. D. *Youth into Maturity.* New York: Mental Health Materials Center, 1970.

ERIKSON, E .H. Identity and the life cycle. *Psychological Issues,* 1:1-171, 1959.

FREUD, S. Analysis, terminable and interminable. In *The Standard Edition of the Complete Psychological Works of Sigmund Freud,* Vol. 23. London: Hogarth Press, 1964, p. 209 (originally published in 1937).

GRINKER, R. R., SR. *Towards a Unified Theory of Human Behavior.* New York: Basic Books, 1956.

GRINKER, R. R. & SPIEGEL, J. *Men under Stress.* Philadelphia: Blakiston, 1945.

GRINKER, R. R., SR. & WERBLE, B. Mentally healthy young males (homoclites): Fourteen years later. *Arch. Gen. Psychiat.,* 30:701-704, 1974.

HARTMAN, E. *Ego Psychology and the Problem of Adaptation.* New York: International Universities Press, 1958.

KAPLAN, A. A philosophical discussion of normality. *Arch. Gen. Psychiat.,* 17:325, 1967.

KING, S. H. Coping mechanisms in adolescents. *Psychiat. Ann.,* 1:10, 1971.

OFFER, D. *The Psychological World of the Teen-ager: A Study of Normal Adolesecnt Boys.* New York: Basic Books, 1973.

OFFER, D., FREEDMAN, D. X., & OFFER, J. The psychiatrist as researcher. In D. Offer & D. X. Freedman (Eds.), *Modern Psychiatry and Clinical Research.* New York: Basic Books, 1972, p. 208.

OFFER, D. & OFFER, J. B. *From Teenage to Young Manhood: A Psychological Study.* New York: Basic Books, Inc., 1975.

OFFER, D., OSTROV, E., & HOWARD, K. I. *The Offer Self-Image Questionnaire for Adolescents.* Chicago: Michael Reese Publication, 1977.

OFFER, D. & SABSHIN, M. *Normality: Theoretical and Clinical Concepts of Mental Health.* New York: Basic Books, 1974.

PETERSEN, A. L., OFFER, D., & SOLOMON, B. *A Study of Normal Adolescent Girls.* Chicago, 1978.

ROMANO, J. Basic orientation and education of the medical student. *J.A.M.A.,* 143: 409, 1950.

ROSENTHAL, D. *Experimenter Effects in Behavioral Research.* New York: Appleton-Century-Crofts, 1966.

SYMONDS, P. M. & JENSEN, A. R. *From Adolescent to Adult.* New York: Columbia University Press, 1961.

VAILLANT, G. E. *Adaptation to Life.* Boston: Little, Brown and Company, 1977.

VON BERTALANFFY, L. *General Systems Theory.* New York: Braziller, 1968.

WELSH, J. B. & OFFER, D. Delinquent self-image and social change. In E. J. Anthony & C. Hiland (Eds.), *The Child in His Family.* New York: John Wiley and Sons, 1978.

WHITE, R. W. *Lives in Progress.* New York: Dryden, 1952.

Part II

EVALUATION AND DIAGNOSIS

Part II takes the reader through the sequential steps of the diagnostic evaluation in adolescent psychiatry. While borrowing from approaches and techniques of child psychiatry on the one hand and of adult psychiatry on the other, the authors nevertheless stress the unique opportunities—and pitfalls—that await the clinician in the evaluation of the adolescent patient.

Allan Z. Schwartzberg, in Chapter 5, stresses the need of the clinician to have knowledge of adolescent development, normal adolescent and family functioning, and adolescent psychopathology. He outlines the steps in the interview with the adolescent and with the family. Clinical examples are used to highlight difficult differential diagnostic problems such as adolescent adjustment reaction, borderline personality, and depression in adolescents.

In *Psychological Testing of Adolescents*, Rebecca E. Rieger describes the multiple ways that psychological testing can contribute to the evaluation of adolescents. Various tests are outlined and their specific utility is reviewed. Through clinical examples, the non-psychologist learns how to get more from psychological testing and to work collaboratively with the psychologist.

In Chapter 7, *The Diagnostic Spectrum in Adolescent Psychiatry: DSM II and DSM III,* Judith L. Rapoport and Rachel Gittelman focus on the concept of the "good diagnosis" in adolescent psychiatry and on changes between The American Psychiatric Association's Diagnostic and Statistical Manual III and its predecessor, DSM II. New diagnostic categories are highlighted.

5

Diagnostic Evaluation of Adolescents

ALLAN Z. SCHWARTZBERG, M.D.

A meaningful approach to diagnosis in adolescent psychiatry must include a knowledge of adolescent development, normal adolescent and family functioning, as well as an adequate knowledge of adolescent psychopathology. In addition to this background, effective psychiatric assessment of the adolescent involves the skill and ability to relate not only to the adolescent but also to his parents.

During the past several decades significant advances have been made in our conceptualization of adolescent development by such authors as Blos (1962), Anna Freud (1969), Erik Erikson (1959), Offer (1969), and many others. They have all greatly enhanced our understanding of adolescent psychodynamics and of the developmental tasks which must be mastered if the adolescent is to proceed successfully toward adulthood.

Anna Freud (1969) has characterized the adolescent period as a "developmental disturbance." She does not feel that adolescent tasks can be acomplished without upheaval in character and personality, since the ego is viewed as having insufficient strength to handle problems. Blos has also described development as involving a profound reorganization of psychiatric structures, a process frequently accompanied by upheaval and chaos. Erikson (1959) has described the major growth task of adolescence as the establishment of a stable ego identity. Ego identity is defined as "both a persistent sameness within oneself (self sameness) and a persistent sharing of some kind of essential character with others" (p. 102). In a major study of a modal group of "normal teenagers" Offer found that the majority of the teenagers in his sample of 73 subjects coped successfully. They lacked the turmoil of disturbed adolescents precisely because their ego was strong enough to withstand the pressures. King (1971) summarized recent studies of healthy adolescents and young adults as follows: 1) The identity crisis is not a common occurrence and the amount of turmoil and conflict is limited; 2) relationships between the adolescent and his parents are generally good; 3) relationships with peers are good; 4) the sense of competence and self-esteem is high; 5) the capacity for coping is high and is achieved by the use of several adaptive mechanisms, including sublimation, a sense of humor and anticipatory planning.

DEFINITION OF ADOLESCENCE

While there are many definitions of adolescence, a 1975 edition of the American Psychiatric Association Psychiatric Glossary presents a definition with broad usefulness: "a chronological period beginning with the physical and emotional processes leading to the sexual and psychosocial maturity and ending at an ill-defined time when the individual achieves independence and social productivity. The period is associated with rapid physical, psychological and social changes." For purposes of conceptualization, diagnosis and treatment, adolescence is arbitrarily divided between the early adolescent phase, ages 12 to 14, mid-adolescence, ages 14 through 17, and late adolescence, ages 18 through 22 (corresponding to the college years).

Early Adolescence

Early adolescence is initiated by puberty with the physiological and hormonal changes such as menses in girls and the appearance of seminal emissions in boys (girls, 12.5 years; boys, 14.5 years). During early adolescence the youngster becomes acquainted with the change in himself and body image and begins to achieve definitive separation and differentiation of the new self from parents. New experimentation with peer relationships of both sexes begins to occur (GAP, 1968). Some of the major characteristics of this phase of adolescent development are as follows: 1) rebellion against and withdrawal from adults and value systems; 2) intense narcissism with the strong preoccupation with one's own body and self; 3) increased importance of the peer group; 4) development and expression of intense sexual urges, thoughts, feelings and fantasies; 5) marked increase in aggressive drives supported by a corresponding increase in physical size and strength; 6) marked increase in emotional and intellectual capabilities with the parallel broadening of interest in activities; and 7) much fluctuation in experimentation, attitudes, and behavior.

Middle Adolescence

During mid-adolescence the teenager must come to terms with a new body image and developing sexual identity. Just as the first phase of adolescence is initiated by increased strength of the intinctual drives, (id impulses), so, too, the second phase of adolescence, beginning roughly in mid-teens, is followed by shift in the balance of forces between the ego and id; in normal development this shift, of course, is in the favor of the ego. This development is associated with an increased capacity for abstract thinking, initiation of dating and increased heterosexual interests, as well as increasing movement towards separation and individuation.

Late Adolescence

The primary tasks of late adolescence are further separation and independence from the family of origin and the development of a firm sense of ego and sexual identity. Additional tasks include the making of a career choice with a commitment to work, the development of a personal moral values system, the capacity for lasting interpersonal relationships and for heterosexual relationships and, finally, a return to the parents with a new relationship based upon relative equality.

It is the purpose of this paper to present a diagnostic approach and method of evaluation for adolescent patients. Diagnosis in adolescence is a dynamic, rather than a static, process, since the adolescent personality is evolving with considerable fluctuation and shifts between id, ego and superego. The clinician should strive for as much understanding and precision as possible in the diagnosis of adolescents, while attempting to avoid labeling. Thus, a term such as chronic schizophrenia should not be used in early adolescence, unless this is process schizophrenia.

Strauss (1975) states, "a psychiatric diagnosis should provide a maximum of useful information for identifying and dealing with a patient's psychiatric condition. It should imply a description of patient's main characteristics and indicate as fully as possible the etiology and prognosis of his disorder and treatment needs" (p. 1193). Recently, attempts to improve the diagnosis of child psychiatric disorders have led to the investigation of a four-axis system involving symptoms, developmental/intellectual level, associated physical condition, and associated psychosocial condition (Rutter et al., 1969). The DSM III (Spitzer and Sheehy, 1976) classification in regard to children's and adolescents' classified disorders on a multi-axial system includes: Axis I. Clinical Psychiatric Syndrome, Axis II. Personality Disorder, Axis III. Nonmental Medical Disorders, Axis IV. Psychosocial Distress, and Axis V. Adaptive Functioning.

RELEVANT LITERATURE FOR ADOLESCENT DIAGNOSTIC EVALUATION

McDonald (1965) reviewed the literature on evaluation in child psychiatry. She noted that Greenacre (1937) had observed "nowhere is there any adequate discussion of the principles of psychiatric examination." McDonald added that "these words written over a quarter of a century ago are applicable today to the entire literature of child psychiatry." She noted that Finch (1960) and Soddy (1960) devoted single brief chapters to descriptions of the diagnostic process but that there was no cohesive discussion of an organized evaluation procedure from dynamic and clinical viewpoints. She observed that Thoma (1933), a German author, stressing thoroughness in child psychiatric evaluation, highlighted areas important for clinical assessment: 1) the potentiality of the ego functioning, 2) the child's conflicts and how he copes with them, 3) the interplay of inhibiting and driving factors, 4) the rigidity and changeability of personality traits and 5) possible directions of development. Thoma's schema bears strong resemblance to the excellent Hampstead Clinic Diagnostic Profile described by Anna Freud (1962).

McDonald stressed repeatedly that her psychiatric method of evaluating children consisted of the following procedures: 1) collecting observations, 2) formulating a diagnostic opinion and recommendation, 3) presenting the results of the diagnostic opinion to the parents and, when indicated, to the child and 4) helping parents and child to take appropriate action upon the recommendation.

Dynamic/genetic formulations in child psychiatric evaluation were discussed thoroughly in a publication by the GAP Committee on Child Psychiatry in 1957 entitled *The Diagnostic Process in Child Psychiatry*. Further elaboration occurred in 1966 with a publication, *The Psychopathological Disorders in Childhood: Theoretical Considerations in a Proposed Classification*. The Accreditation Manual for Psychiatric Facilities Serving Children and Adolescents, (APA, 1971) stresses the importance of a variety of diagnosis and treatment plans in inpatient facilities, such as physical, psychological, developmental, chronological, familial, educational, social, environmental, and recreational. In recent years, Meeks (1971), in his book, *The Fragile Alliance,* presented a chapter on the diagnostic evaluation of adolescents. Recent authors writing on child and adolescent diagnostic evaluation include Werkman (1965), Cohen (1976), and Haslett (1977).

DIAGNOSTIC CONSIDERATIONS

Many adolescents are brought to the psychiatrist's office not only because of unresolved tasks of childhood development but also because of conflicts precipitated by the onset of adolescence itself. The approach to the adolescent must, therefore, be developmental. The following basic questions need to be considered in the assessment of the adolescent at any age: 1) What is the highest level of psychosocial development? 2) What is the quality of family relationships, especially with the parents? 3) What is the quality of the interpersonal and peer relationships? 4) What is the level of school interest, involvement, and academic performance? 5) What are the adolescent's extracurricular interests and activities? 6) Are there pathological indicators such as self-destructive, antisocial, acting-out, or bizarre behavior? 7) Is there a significant conflict requiring psychotherapeutic intervention? 8) If psychotherapy is indicated, does the adolescent have the capacity and interest in observing himself (observing ego) and the motivation to enter into a therapeutic alliance with the therapist? 9) Is the family's attitude toward the psychotherapist's treatment constructive, encouraging autonomy, or resistant to change and likely to sabotage the treatment process? 10) What are the adolescent's strengths and assets?

INITIATING THE DIAGNOSTIC EVALUATION

Whenever possible, the initial contact should be with the adolescent. If the parents call for an appointment and if the adolescent is available, the psychiatrist should request to talk with the adolescent directly to make the appointment. Older adolescents are far more likely to request independent psychiatric evaluation and to make their own appointment. When it is not possible to speak with the adolescent, due to either unavailability of the adolescent or marked resistance, an appointment is made with the parents. This not only allows for assessment of the presenting problem and the parental attitude toward the problem, but also enables the clinician to secure valuable background information and to have the opportunity to enlist parents as allies in the evaluation process and potentially in treatment.

The psychiatrist should keep foremost in his mind the desire to appeal to the independent, autonomous part of the adolescent's ego so that the whole evaluation process becomes growth-promoting. When the initial appointment is with the parents, it should be stressed over the telephone that *both parents* should be present for the initial interview. This allows the therapist to perceive the similarities and differences between the mother's and the father's perceptions of the adolescent's problem. The interview may readily highlight a marital problem smouldering beneath the surface. The psychiatrist is careful both to observe and elicit patterns of coalition, defenses, and communication, not only between parent and child, but between the parents themselves. If there are older children, it is useful to ask about their status and see how well they have coped during the adolescent period.

FAMILY ASSESSMENT

Research on Family Systems

In assessing the adolescent's family, the psychiatrist should have some awareness of recent research findings on family systems and incorporate this knowledge into his thinking and practice. Westley and Epstein (1969) noted that successful families were characterized by: 1) successful problem-solving, 2) effective communication with clear, direct messages sent, 3) healthy affective interaction among all family members with special emphasis on empathic interaction between parent and child and between husband and wife, 4) effective role and power allocations, and 5) effective granting of autonomy to adolescents.

More recently, Lewis, Beavers, Gossett and Phillips (1976), extending the original work of Westley, have noted five parameters necessary for the development of capable, healthy, adaptive individuals: 1) Leadership is shared between the parents, changing with the nature of the interaction. 2) There is a strong parental coalition. 3) There is closeness in the family but with distinct individuation and boundaries among members. 4) The power structure is easy to determine through efficient problem-solving. 5) There is clear communication, with members voicing responsibility for individual actions; there is a lack of evasiveness or "mindreading" statements. Open, direct expression of feelings, with minimal conflict and maximum empathic responsiveness, is present.

Beavers and Lewis (1975) classified adolescent pathology into four groups: healthy, neurotic, behavior disorder, and psychotic. A clinical rating scale indicated differences between mid-range families (i.e. families with neurotic and behavior disorder children) and extreme groups (i.e. healthy and psychotic), as well as differences between the two types of mid-range families. In mid-range families: 1) separation-individuation is successful; 2) ambivalence, anger, and sexuality are viewed with disdain; 3) an abstract code of morality —often personified in a particular person such as a grandparent or a legislator—is adhered to; 4) a rigid rule system is adopted that often leads to scapegoating; 5) the rigidity resulting from the tight rule system often leads to power struggless between parents.

Neurotic and behavior disordered families are distinguished in the following ways: 1) Both family types adhered to rigid authoritarian rule. In the neurotic group the parents form a coalition to maintain and enforce family rules in such a way that one spouse is dominant and the other subservient. In the behavior disorder group the need for adherence to a highly structured family system is the same, but there is no parental coalition to maintain it. 2) The neurotic family uses repression to rid itself of unacceptable feelings and thoughts, as prescribed by the moral code. In the behavior disorder family, denial and projection are used but frequently such defenses are ineffective and open rule-breaking occurs. 3) Behavior disorder families display frequent crises which often serve to maintain equilibrium by pointing to an increased need to control and restrict impulses.

The psychotic family is frequently leaderless and amorphous regarding individual boundaries and severely conflict ridden.

The Family Interview

It is best at the outset to explain the entire diagnostic procedure after establishing rapport with parents. It should be explained that there will be one or more meetings with the adolescent, that confidentiality needs to be respected, that there subsequently will be a joint family interview followed by psychological testing if necessary, and that, finally, there will be a post-diagnostic session which involves review of the clinical interviews, results of testing, summarization and recommendation. The purpose of the interview should be clearly stated and cooperation elicited so that observable data may be gathered to help truly understand the adolescent in a comprehensive way. Many parents are relieved when they are aware of the evaluation process and feel that the psychiatrist has a sense of purpose and direction and is "captain of the team" in this process.

During the initial interview with parents it is useful to obtain some of the following information: the presenting problem (such as school underachievement, depression, or acting-out behavior); the onset of the symptoms, their duration, severity, and course; the precipitating factors; the family's attitude toward the presenting problem; the family's own assessment of etiological factors; efforts and result of prior help from family physicians, schools, and psychotherapists. It is best to try to record presenting problems in the parents' own words in a few sentences such as "He's been doing poorly in school and seems to have no friends." The psychiatrist's assessment of the parents' feelings and attitudes toward the problems provides additional valuable data.

Additional areas in history-taking relate to perinatal history, medical history with developmental milestones, family history, school history, and assessment of the child's strengths and assets, as well as use of his leisure time. Evaluation of the developmental history should include normal developmental milestones (with factors surrounding pregnancy and childbirth) ; normal milestones for sitting up, walking, talking, etc.; evidence of eating disorders or disturbances in toilet training; early socialization responses in nursery school; and response to separation from parents in kindergarten. Similarly, each developmental stage should be assessed in turn. The psychiatrist should note trends and patterns of school interests and academic performance, as well as outside interests. Special attention should be given to how the adolescent has coped during transitional periods such as leaving elementary school, junior high school, and high school. If there has been a delay or difficulty in mastering a developmental phase, further questioning is necessary. If psychotherapeutic intervention has been required, what has been the response?

The psychiatrist needs to ascertain the parents' perception of the adolescent's interests, hobbies, extracurricular activities, future plans and goal direction, as well as attitudes toward peers and the peer group. If there has been evidence of drug use, the psychiatrist should inquire about the pattern, trend and frequency, use of hard drugs, and the parents' attitudes toward drugs, as well as toward acting-out behavior in general.

Certainly not all these questions will be necessary for all parents or adolescents in any given interview. When the problem area is identified, however, the psychiatrist should attempt to go into as much depth as possible to obtain a clear picture of the presenting problem.

Parents often ask, "How can I get my teenager to your office when he doesn't want to come?" It helps greatly for the clinician to assist the parents in conceptualizing the problem as a family problem which needs solution. A parent might say, "We're all in this together. Let's find out if there's a problem. Let's see why we're having so much difficulty talking with each other." In the majority of instances, when this approach is taken and when the parents are united on the need for an evaluation, the adolescent, despite some complaining, will go along with psychiatric consultation. If the adolescent threatens to come and not talk, the parents should not be intimidated but should say, "Let's keep an open mind. Let's get an expert's opinion." While most referrals are initiated by parents, self-referrals, especially by older adolescents, can be especially productive since these adolescents are often sufficiently anxious, motivated and "ready to work."

INTERVIEW WITH THE ADOLESCENT

The psychiatrist's task in the initial interview is to create a sufficiently warm emotional climate to enable the adolescent to talk freely and unburden himself. The purpose of the interview is not only to try to understand the adolescent and why he comes for evaluation at this patricular point in time, but also to collect behavioral observations, to relieve anxiety, to establish rapport and to overcome initial resistance. This is not an easy task, especially for early adolescents or acting-out and very negativistic teenagers who feel coerced into coming for the interview. It is important to recognize that high levels of anxiety occur with most initial interviews. Reactions often range from overt hostility and negativism to sullenness, withdrawal, silence, and surface compliance. It is the psychiatrist's job first and foremost to relieve anxiety and deal with initial resistances to evaluation. Where the adolescent manifests marked initial resistance or even refuses to be seen separately, an initial family interview, as outlined above, is often helpful to define the nature and purpose of the evaluation.

Flexibility of approach is essential. Following the family interview during the first part of the initial session, an interview with the adolescent is often quite productive. Information may be obtained regarding the immediate feelings during the family interview. The clinician can note not only verbal patterns of interaction but also nonverbal behavior, particularly seating arrangement and body language such as posture, voice tone, facial expression, eye contact, etc.

After the initial contact, the adolescent may be asked neutral questions in an effort to further relieve anxiety and foster rapport. These questions may relate to where he goes to school, favorite subjects, sports, extracurricular activities, favorite TV programs, etc. When the adolescent's anxiety is further reduced, the psychiatrist needs to inquire about the adolescent's feelings and reactions to the evaluation interview. Was he informed? How did he feel about coming? What were his feelings immediately during the family session? Does he feel there is a problem? If so, how does he define it? If the adolescent begins to blame the parents, the therapist should encourage him to relate the story with as few interruptions as possible rather than challenging him. A friendly interest leads to empathic, responsive listening, which is useful in encouraging the adolescent to continue. Sincere human interest conveyed allows him to further elaborate his story. Measured activity and flexibility are important principles, avoiding, on the one hand, analytic detachment and, on the other hand, excessive questioning, which may be perceived as too threatening or controlling.

Additional principles of interviewing of the adolescent include sensitivity, establishment of rapport and confidentiality, and empathic listening. The psychiatrist may alternate between being the objective understanding adult and identifying with the teenager in an attempt to see how the adolescent sees the world. It is important to keep the conversation flowing and not to allow long silences which help to generate intense anxiety. In general, silences are more easily tolerated by adults; they may be experienced by the adolescent as rejection, thus increasing resistance to the evaluation process.

Confidentiality

After the initial neutral questions, the adolescent should be informed that the interview is confidential, that he should be able to talk without fear of retaliation or recriminations. It should be explained, however, that there are limits to confidentiality when, in the therapist's judgment, the adolescent's behavior is dangerous and life-threatening either to himself or to others. It should be stressed that when communications occur with the parents in ongoing treatment, the psychiatrist will not betray the adolescent's confidence though he will feel free to discuss the information conveyed to him by parents with the adolescent.

A pattern of very frequent drug use combined with acting-out behavior will surely test the psychiatrist's efforts to maintain confidentiality. It should be explained that the psychiatrist will exercise his best judgment and, in fact, may well have to revise the original treatment plan if and when circumstances dictate the need for hospitalization or specialized treatment programs. In these situations, parent involvement and cooperation are crucial.

Dealing with Resistance

Many adolescents, especially early adolescents, display strong defenses of denial, negativism, and silence during the initial interview. They are embarrassed, anxious, and angry about consultation and they view the entire procedure as a conspiracy among adults to "gang up" on them. The psychiatrist needs to be aware of these defenses and to try to overcome them as quickly as possible. As stated previously, after some neutral questions have been asked and initial anxiety dissipated, the clinician might proceed as follows: "As you know, your parents have contacted me and mentioned some of their concerns to me about you. I would like to try to understand the situation. Just what do you think they're worried about?" An attitude which attempts to understand the adolescent through sincere empathy and interest can go a long way towards reassuring him and relieving anxiety.

Once anxiety is sufficiently relieved, the psychiatrist wants to find out the adolescent's own view of the presenting problem, which may be school underachievement, truancy, depression, lack of friends, etc. Are the defenses of both denial and projection maintained or can the adolescent acknowledge and reveal any personal problems and take responsibility for his own actions? As the interview progresses further, one should attempt to assess immediate areas of dysfunction through such questions as, "Tell me about your family. How do people relate to each other? How do you feel you get along with your parents and siblings? Who do you seem to have the most conflict with? How have you been feeling lately? Do you see any relationship between your symptoms (e.g. depression) and conflict with your parents?" The clinician should attempt to have as clear a picture as possible of family dynamics and interactions and the role which the adolescent plays within the family. Is there an alternate game of victim-persecutor? It is particularly important to get his impression of his family's problem-solving ability, communication patterns, defenses, and affective interactions. How the parents relate to each other and patterns of sharing of power, e.g., dominance and submission, are of crucial importance.

Peer Relationships

In the area of peer relationships, the therapist should ask about preferred activities and the number of friends, carefully distinguishing between "acquaintances" and real friends. An excellent question to ask is what the adolescent most prefers to do after school and on weekends and which peers are preferred for these activities. Such a question reveals a good deal about the adolescent's ability to sublimate drive energies. Are there sublimated interests or is there a good deal of idleness, boredom, loneliness, and withdrawal? Are friendships stable and supportive or are they fleeting and ephemeral? For mid-adolescents, it is useful to ask about experience and comfort in dating relationships and, where indicated, sexual involvement. A very useful approach is to ask the adolescent to describe his best friend, what is most and least likable about this person and, conversely, his best friend's perception of him. Valuable information can be gained about the mirrored narcissistic image that is self-reflected in the choice of a best friend, as well as the friend's range of interests and activities.

School

In regard to school, it is important to ascertain the adolescent's level of school interest and performance. It is important to learn his attitudes toward school: Is he curious and eager for learning or does he show a pattern of underachievement, boredom, and procrastination? Intellectual abilities may be grossly estimated not only from preliminary information conveyed by parents but also from the adolescent's vocabulary, range of interests, alertness, and speed of response during the interview. Further assessment of attitudes towards school may be obtained through questions regarding his relationships with teachers in general, his favorite teachers and subjects, his relationship with peers within the school, and the degree of interest and involvement in extracurricular activities.

Self Observation

Toward the end of the initial interview it is important to arouse interest and curiosity about the self. Are there any areas about himself or his family situation that he would like to see changed? If so, is he willing to put forth the necessary effort involved in effecting change? Does he think his family will become involved as needed in the treatment process? How much responsibility is he assuming for his current dilemma? What types of symptoms is he experiencing and with what severity?

It is important throughout the interview to try to gauge the level and intensity of anxiety, depression, withdrawal, pattern of concentration, disturbance in thinking and comprehension. If the adolescent acknowledges depression, it is mandatory to ask about suicidal ideation, plans and history of previous attempts; in general, the psychiatrist and the adolescent should assess, to their satisfaction, the seriousness of suicidal intent. If there are antisocial, acting-out behavior patterns, has the adolescent been in trouble with the law, is he involved with drugs and, if so, to what extent? Has he come to rely on them? A pattern of heavy drug use and depression should elicit further questions about runaway fantasies or experiences. Eliciting runaway fantasies can provide an underlying clue to magical rescue fantasies. If the adolescent has run away before, what actually occurred and how did the parents respond? Additional useful questions relate to patterns of sexual promiscuity and exploitation in relationships with both sexes. Another useful approach is to ask the adolescent what three wishes he most would like for himself, thus providing a clue to underlying deep wishes, needs, conflict areas, and potential solutions to these conflicts. All adolescents, especially late adolescents, have real concern about career aspirations and college choices. Questions in these areas are often perceived as signs of friendly interest.

Closing the Initial Interview

If there has been a history of prior psychiatric treatment, the psychiatrist should inquire about the results. Toward the end of the initial interview, he should try to obtain the adolescent's cooperation to continue the evaluation procedure. When rapport has developed and the adolescent has been "engaged," he will readily agree to return for an additional interview. If the adolescent has been seen first and he is living at home, the clinician should explain that a family interview is usually very helpful in understanding his history and his current conflicts. While there may be initial resistance to the family interview, it helps greatly to reassure the adolescent that confidentiality will be respected, that appropriate support will be present, and that every effort will be made to provide an atmosphere of openness, flexibility, and mutual respect.

When psychological testing is indicated, e.g., to assess psychodynamics, organicity, or precise intellectual functioning, it is helpful to indicate to the adolescent that psychological testing provides a more complete picture of his current personality functioning. The nature of the psychological tests should be explained. Where rapport is established and cooperation is obtained, the therapist should indicate that these tests, along with the results of the interviews, will be reviewed with the adolescent and his family at a post-diagnostic session. It should be stated that psychological tests can help provide a "blueprint" to understand precisely the nature of his problem in order to shorten the whole time period for the psychotherapeutic process.

Close cooperation between psychiatrist and testing psychologist is essential. The clinician should want to know the following information: What type of personality is evolving? What are the adolescent's core conflicts? What defenses are being utilized and to what degree of success? What is the overall clinical impression? In addition to asking about areas of core conflict and psychodynamics, the clinician needs to know about the evidences of ego strength, assets, healthy ego functioning, and the prognosis with and without psychotherapeutic intervention.

SUMMARY OF ADOLESCENT AND
PARENT INTERVIEWS

Following interviews with the adolescent individually and with the parents, it is important to integrate the clinical observations and psychological test data into an integrated formulation. The formulation should take into account not only the data from clinical interviews and psychological testing, but also (when indicated) information from schools, medical reports, previous psychological testing and/or psychiatric treatment reports. Psychosocial, cultural, physical factors, in addition to psychodynamic considerations, should all be taken into account.

McDonald (1965) states that the diagnostic formulation must include an assessment of: a) the child's conflicts, b) the child's personality and developmental progress, c) constitutional factors, i.e., organic impairments and major psychological traumas, and d) parents' role in the child's external world. She concludes that the psychiatrist has to be clear about what he knows and does not know and about what confuses him. Only then is he ready for the follow-up interview. Formulation should include a summary statement regarding what is known about intrapsychic and interpersonal dynamics and with a summary of major defenses utilized by both the family and the adolescent in their observed interactions.

FOLLOW-UP INTERVIEW

The post-diagnostic or follow-up interview is the culmination of all the evaluation efforts to date. This allows integration of all previous data gathered from parents, the adolescent, family interviews, psychological test data, school and medical reports, etc. This conference, which the family and the adolescent have been anxiously awaiting, presents a real challenge to the psychiatrist. His task is to integrate the data acquired into a meaningful diagnosis from clinical, dynamic, and genetic viewpoints, and to make optimal recommendations, not only for the adolescent but also for his family. Haslett (1977) recommends that treatment plans be outlined in writing, with specific objectives, strategies, and the estimated length of time that psychotherapeutic intervention will be required. It is important to try to be as specific as possible in terms of both the diagnostic formulation and treatment recommendations.

Wherever possible, the adolescent and the parents should be seen together for the post-diagnostic follow-up session. When there is strong resistance to joint interview, seeing the parents and adolescent separately often allows for securing cooperation for treatment plans, reducing anxiety, and encouraging motivation for treatment. Utilizing the rapport established in previous interviews, the psychiatrist should try to present his treatment recommendations as clearly and as simply as possible to the individual adolescent and to the family group. A few essential points should be highlighted relating to both diagnosis and recommendations.

During the post-diagnostic interview the psychiatrist should attempt to elucidate one of the five possible goals for therapeutic intervention (GAP, 1973) : 1) intrapsychic modification, 2) alteration of intrafamilial functioning, 3) alteration of peer group interaction, 4) modification of adolescent school or community adjustment, or 5) removal of the adolescent from the family with placement in a different environment, i.e., hospitalization or residential treatment. Often these goals are not mutually exclusive but overlapping; hence, recommendations are made for combined modalities and treatment.

Clinical judgment and the timing of recommendations are of crucial importance. The clinician should present his recommendations with conviction in order to get agreement on a therapeutic contract. When individual psychotherapy is recommended, it should be explained that conjoint family interviews will also be necessary on either a regular or a periodic basis.

COMMON PSYCHIATRIC SYNDROMES

Adolescent Adjustment Reactions

One of the commonest diagnoses is that of Adolescent Adjustment Reaction, a term which is used much too often with too little precision. It is considered by many to be a wastebasket term. The fact is that, when properly utilized, it may have usefulness and relevance not only for diagnosis but for treatment.

The American Psychiatric Association *Diagnostic and Statistical Manual of Mental Disorders (DSM II)* (APA, 1968) lists the Adjustment Reaction of Adolescence under Transient Situational Personality Disorders, which are defined as, "Those transient disorders of any severity including those of psychotic proportions that occur in individuals without any apparent underlying mental disorders and that represent an acute reaction to overwhelming environmental stress." The manifestations of an adjustment reaction vary with the phase of adolescence and the stresses peculiar to that phase.

The impact of adolescence itself on an individual can be a stress which can cause the adolescent to become emotionally ill for a transient period of time. It is important to distinguish adolescent symptoms from "growing pains" occurring at transitional phases of the adolescent experience. Blaine (1971) notes, "All of the symptoms of emotional illness may appear in lesser degree as idiosyncracies in normal adolescents. Anxiety, depression, hypomanic behavior, drug abuse, stealing, and even temporary breaks with reality can all occur within the context of normality; but when these personality traits become dominant or progress to the point of serious adaptive disruption, they become part of an illness."

In early adolescence the inability to cope may reveal itself in increased irritability, open hostility toward authority figures, or angry temperamental outbursts which are disproportionate to the precipitating circumstances. Some of the stresses of the early adolescence include physiological and hormonal changes of puberty, increased peer pressure to be popular socially and to compete athletically, and increased academic demands. The adolescent may alternate between irritability and aggressive acting-out behavior and withdrawal, passivity, and depression.

In mid-adolescence, episodes of depression, marked anxiety, or regressive behavior may be associated with the increasing need to separate and individuate, increased demands to establish heterosexual relationships, increasing academic demands, and concerns about sexual adequacy and a sense of belonging to a group.

In late adolescence the most common form of adolescent adjustment reaction occurs in the form of the well-known identity crisis. Often the adolescent begins to question, "Who am I? What will become of me? Where am I going?" The late adolescent may experience considerable stress in moving from a comfortable and secure home environment where he has received considerable recognition and security to a college environment which offers little support and intense academic competition. He may experience increased stress in terms of needing to choose a career, needing to have a sense of belonging to a group, and needing to feel comfortable with the opposite sex in a close relationship.

Adolescent adjustment reactions must be differentiated from other clinical conditions occurring during this period. Often the adolescent must be observed over time in order for the diagnosis to become clear. It is important to realize that a diagnosis during the adolescent period is never static but always dynamic. One should attempt to visualize adolescent personality as it evolves and as characterological patterns change and crystallize, especially in late adolescence. Diagnosis must include differentiation of the adolescent adjustment reaction from depression, schizophrenia, character disorders, and borderline personality disorders.

One of the most difficult tasks for the psychiatrist is distinguishing between severe adolescent adjustment reactions and schizophrenia. Often the clinical picture will evolve gradually. For example, Grinker and Holzman (1973), found that one-third of hospitalized adolescents eventually given the diagnosis of schizophrenia presented no diagnostic difficulty. The other two-thirds, however, presented a clinical picture of adolescent adjustment reaction, often with chaos and turmoil states so severe as to be considered of near psychotic proportion. Close observation during the hospitalization of these adolescents revealed basic underlying schizophrenic process.

Case Report

A 19-year-old girl entered psychotherapy because of feelings of anxiety, fluctuating depression, self-doubt, and loss of goal direction. She was the only child of a compulsive, domineering father and rather passive, retiring mother; nevertheless she had felt quite successful socially and academically during her high school years. She was an excellent student with a broad range of interests. After an exhaustive study of colleges, she finally chose to attend a conservative state university rather than a prestgious private college to which she had been accepted. She acknowledged considerable self-doubt about being able to achieve in an "intense" environment.

During her first semester she experienced some acute and fluctuating feelings of depression associated not only with separation from the security of her family but also with finding that she was no longer the center of attention as she had been in the nuclear family and in high school. She became progressively disillusioned with both her loss of supports and her loss of specialness. Short-term psychotherapy enabled her to complete the year, but she decided not to return to the state university.

When she worked during the summer as a camp counselor, she noted a good deal of difficulty in establishing herself as an authority figure. She stated, "I just couldn't control the kids.

My self-esteem and self-confidence just got lower and lower."
She thus suffered two narcissistic injuries within a short time.
As fall approached and she again considered college, she felt
unable to decide to attend her second choice school, fearful that
she might be making a mistake. In reality she seemed fearful
of separating.

No significant psychological difficulty was evident prior to
attending college. Under the impact of separation anxiety, however, she experienced considerable uncertainty, associated with
lowered self-esteem and self-concept. She remarked, "I don't
know my direction anymore. I've been feeling very insecure
about being myself. I find myself sleeping, reading, eating, and
withdrawing. I don't like myself."

She acknowledged confusion, self-doubt and uncertainty about
her identity and direction. A diagnosis was made of an adolescent adjustment reaction in a young woman with an obsessive-
compulsive personality. She had many ego assets. A recommendation for individual and group psychotherapy was accepted.
The patient responded with marked improvement over a six-
month period. With the loss of depressive symptoms and development of a stronger ego identity and direction, she returned
to college and took pleasure in social and academic achievements.

Adolescent Depression

Depression is one of the most common types of reactions in adolescence. This syndrome may be of clinical or subclinical proportions and is associated with the developmental changes concurrent
with separation-individuation. Depression in adolescence may be a
transient, situational disturbance or may develop into a chronic long-
standing state with signs and symptoms similar to those seen in
adult depression.

Depression may occur with schizophrenia, personality disorders,
borderline states, anorexia, as well as in cases of alcohol and drug
use. Depressive symptoms may be associated with difficulty in concentration, crying spells, insomnia, or anorexia. Frequently there is
even a paradoxical increased appetite. Additional symptoms include
social isolation and withdrawal, antisocial, acting-out behavior, and
poor academic performance.

Lorand (1967) has observed that depression in adolescence is
closely related to the detachment from parental authority. The de-

tachment is experienced by the depressed adolescent not as liberation but as abandonment by those objects on whom there has been reliance for guidance and support. Lorand views adolescent depression as similar dynamically to adult depression, which is also related to both the loved and hated object. Additionally, the adolescent feels forced by his superego to change and comply with new demands to relinquish old attachments and form new ones. The ego rebels against these demands and, unable to express aggression, is overwhelmed by feelings of helplessness, with fervent desires to regress to an earlier, less conflict-ridden state of development.

Nicholi (1978) has stated that depression is by far the most frequent and most significant casual factor in the decision to leave college. In a study of college dropouts he found that the student's depression seemed to be closely related to a discrepancy between the actual and ideal states of the self. Awareness of this discrepancy, of failure to attain idealized goals, often resulted in feelings of inadequacy, despair, hopelessness, low self-esteem, self-reproach, and inability to concentrate.

Case Report

A 17-year-old girl was seen for psychiatric evaluation because of frequent crying spells, persistent mood depression, generalized loss of confidence and seclusiveness. A bright girl, she had graduated from high school six months earlier but was continuing to take a few advanced high school courses since she was fearful of attending college. She had obtained a part-time job, but otherwise was largely homebound.

Psychiatric examination revealed a severely constricted, tearful, overtly depressed young woman who remarked, "It seems all right if I were sitting around the house doing nothing for the rest of my life." She went on to relate that she often felt inferior, had no close friends, had never dated, and had never felt part of a group. Simultaneously, she acknowledged that she often felt critical and negativistic toward others while, at the same time, she was very self-conscious. While she was able to relate to some degree to her mother, she remarked that her father, a professor, was always reading the newspaper, watching TV, or trying to lecture her. "I always feel he is trying to teach me a lesson." A budding interest in the media was floundering since her father had repeatedly "criticized her choice of subjects." But the patient was failing computer math, a subject suggested by the father. While there was no evidence of suicidal intent or psychotic thought content, it was clear that she was severely depressed.

After the initial interview with the adolescent, the parents were seen. They acknowledged high academic standards and expectations. The professor-father, an admitted compulsive perfectionist, attempted to openly control the interview. The mother joined the father in her criticism of the patient, being annoyed at the daughter's isolation and procrastination. Both parents were critical of their daughter for barely finishing in the upper third of the class despite a very superior IQ. An overachieving sister, two years older, was openly hypercritical. The patient clearly functioned as the family "lightning rod," absorbing all tensions in the family system.

A diagnosis of severe neurotic depression reaction was made. Reluctantly, the family agreed to a recommendation of both intensive individual psychotherapy and family therapy.

Borderline Personality

Increasingly, the diagnosis of borderline personality is made in adolescence. Writings of Mahler (1971), Kernberg (1976), and Masterson (1972) have given fresh understanding to this disorder with relevance for treatment. Diagnosis of the borderline personality in adolescence presents a formidable diagnostic challenge. Kernberg has proposed the following criteria: 1) There is identity diffusion, i.e. the lack of an integrated concept of self and concept of significant others (self and object representations); 2) Primitive defensive constellations, centering around splitting predominate. He feels that these two criteria differentiate borderline conditions from symptomatic neuroses and non-borderline character pathology, all of which present a solid ego identity in a predominance of defensive mechanisms centering around repression. 3) Reality testing is maintained. Reality testing is evaluated in three successive steps by: a) evaluating the presence or absence of true hallucinations and delusions; b) evaluating the patient's capacity to empathize with the interviewer's observations regarding strange or bizarre aspects of the patient's behavior, affect, or thought content in the here and now; and c) evaluating the consequences of interpretation of primitive defensive operations in the patient-therapist observation.

Gunderson and Singer (1975) have proposed criteria for borderline patients which involve affects, behavior, psychotic episodes or regression under stress, psychological test performance, and interpersonal relations. Borderline adolescents might appear hostile, display acting-out of anger, or even have rage reactions. The anger may be directed inwardly or externally. Depressive loneliness may be present along with a pervading sense of futility. Characteristically, there is poor impulse control and suicidal threats and/or attempts. Brief psychotic episodes, which are usually transient and reversible, may occur under stress. Disorted thought processes are revealed, especially on projective tests such as the Rorschach. There is a tendency to reason circumstantially rather than logically, as well as a tendency to read more affective elaboration into perceptions than normally. Finally, interpersonal relationships are characteristically superficial and transient, lacking real emotional depth and responsiveness. The patient experiences difficulty with close emotional relationships and frequently develops a manipulative and devaluative stance toward others in a very demanding fashion.

Case Report

A 22-year-old woman came for psychotherapy with a long psychiatric history. She presented a long history of separation problems, beginning, with partial regression at age 15 months when a sister was born. She could not continue in nursery school after one month. Separation anxiety continued in kindergarten and the first grade. After a relatively quiescent period during elementary school, she again experienced separation anxiety while attending junior high school, resulting in progressive withdrawal. Psychotherapy on a weekly basis was undertaken without success. By mid teens, however, she had refused to go to school and had socially and emotionally isolated herself. She finally was referred to a residential treatment program which she attended two years. Following her return to her home, she attended college but continued to be socially isolated and constricted.

Over the years this young woman had developed and maintained an alienated hostile relationship with all of her family members. She was noted to have an especially hostile and dependent relationship with her mother. She had never been able to form any peer relationships and had never had any dating relationships. Reports from her residential treatment center indicated that she did a good deal of complaining and perceived the world as being divided into black and white, with herself being good and the rest of the world evil. She complained repeatedly that everyone was inconsiderate of her and no one liked her; on the other hand she did not care much for anybody else either. The only affect displayed was tremendous rage. It was noted that she displayed "as if" behavior, often behaving as she was expected to behave. For example, she spoke of watching herself "take part in a play in which only I know it's an act to please others."

During initial psychiatric examination, she described depression, anger, mood swings, and concern that a beginning relationship with a boy was causing her distress. She acknowledged "fear of getting physically close and fear of trusting." She presented herself as frightened, sullen, hostile and distant with poorly concealed anger. She stated, "I feel confused. I don't know who I am or where I am. I don't know what I want." While there was no overt suicidal intent, she acknowledged chronic fluctuating depression.

Her only source of warmth was a pet dog acquired during her stay at the treatment center. There was no evidence of overt psychosis. Previous clinical diagnoses included "ambulatory schizophrenic reaction, mixed neurotic reaction, chronic character disorder, with paranoid tendencies, paranoid personality, schizoid personality. The clinical impression was that she was presenting with a borderline personality organization. Despite extensive previous psychotherapy, further intensive individual psychotherapy was recommended.

SUMMARY

This chapter has presented a diagnostic approach and method of psychiatric evaluation for the adolescent patient. The different phases of adolescent development and their implications for diagnosis have been stressed throughout. Important diagnostic questions have been raised regarding highest level of development and quality of family, school and social functioning, along with extracurricular interests and evidence of pathological indicators.

The importance of a flexible, open approach with adolescents, as well as the need to adequately assess the family system, has been stressed. Dealing effectively with early resistances and establishing therapeutic rapport, confidentiality and a therapeutic working alliance have been emphasized. Methods for handling post-diagnostic or follow-up interview and recommendations have been presented. Finally, clinical examples have been presented of some of the commonest types of adolescent problems, including the adolescent adjustment reaction, depression, schizophrenia and borderline personality.

REFERENCES

AMERICAN PSYCHIATRIC ASSOCIATION. *A Psychiatric Glossary.* Washington, D. C., 1975.
AMERICAN PSYCHIATRIC ASSOCIATION. *Diagnostic and Statistical Manual of Mental Disorders (D.S.M. II).* Washington, D. C., 1968.
AMERICAN PSYCHIATRIC ASSOCIATION. *Standards for Psychiatric Facilities Serving Children and Adolescents.* Washington, D. C., 1971, pp. 30-32.
BEAVERS, W. R. & LEWIS, J. Family systems in individual functioning. Mid-range families. Read before American Psychiatric Association meeting in Anaheim, California, May, 1975.
BLAINE, G. Adjustment reaction of adolescents. *Psychiatric Annals,* 3:46-71, 1971.
BLOS, P. *On Adolescence.* Glencoe, Illinois: The Free Press, 1962,, p. 73.
COHEN, D. The diagnostic process of child psychiatry. *Psychiatric Annals,* 6(9):29-56, 1976.
ERIKSON, E. Identity and the life cycle. *Psychol. Issues,* 1:1, Monog. 1. New York: International Universities Press, 1959.
FINCH, S. M. *Fundamentals of Child Psychiatry.* New York: Norton, 1960.
FREUD, A. Adolescence as a developmental disturbance. In G. Kaplan & S. Lebovici (Eds.), *Adolescence: Psychosocial Perspectives.* New York: Basic Books, 1969.
FREUD, A. Assessment of childhood disturbances. In *The Psychoanalytic Study of the Child,* 17:149-158. New York: International Universities Press, 1962.
GREENACRE, P. Review of practical examination of personality and behavior disorders. *Psychoanal. Quart.,* 6:134, 1937.
GRINKER, R., SR. & HOLZMAN, P. Schizophrenic pathology in young adults. *Arch. Gen. Psychiat.,* 28:168-175, 1973.
GROUP FOR THE ADVANCEMENT OF PSYCHIATRY, COMMITTEE ON CHILD PSYCHIATRY. *The Diagnostic Process of Child Psychiatry.* GAP Report, No. 38. New York, 1957.
GROUP FOR THE ADVANCEMENT OF PSYCHIATRY, COMMITTEE ON CHILD PSYCHIATRY. *Psychopathological Disorders in Childhood: Theoretical Considerations and a Proposed Classification,* Volume 6. GAP Report No. 62. New York, 1966.
GROUP FOR THE ADVANCEMENT OF PSYCHIATRY. *From Diagnosis to Treatment: An Approach to Treatment Planning for the Emotionally Disturbed Child,* Volume 8. GAP Report No. 87. New York, 1973.
GROUP FOR THE ADVANCEMENT OF PSYCHIATRY. *Normal Adolescence.* New York: Charles Scribner and Sons, 1968, pp. 59-93.
GUNDERSON, J. & SINGER, M. Defining borderline patients: An overview. *American Journal of Psychiatry,* 132:1-10, 1975.
HASLETT, N. Treatment and planning for children: The complete childhood psychiatry evaluation outline. *J. Contin. Educ. Psychiat.,* 21-34, 1977.
KERNBERG, O. *Borderline Conditions and Pathological Narcissism.* New York: Aronson, 1975.
KERNBERG, O. *Object-Relations Theory in Clinical Psychoanalysis.* New York: Aronson, 1976.
KING, S. H. Coping mechanisms in adolescence. *Psychiat. Ann.,* 1(3):46, Nov. 1971.
LEWIS, J. M., BEAVERS, W. R., GOSSETT, J. T., & PHILLIPS, V. A. *No Single Thread: Psychological Health in Family Systems.* New York: Brunner/Mazel, 1976.

LORAND, S. Adolescent depression. *Int. J. Psychoanal.*, 48:53-60, 1967.

MAHLER, M. The study of the separation-individuation process and its possible application to borderline phenomenon in the psychoanalytic situation. *Psychoanal. Study Child.*, 26:403-425, 1971.

MASTERSON, J. *Treatment of the Borderline Adolescent: A Developmental Approach.* New York: Wiley-Interscience, 1972.

McDONALD, M. Psychiatric evaluation in children. *J. Acad. Child Psychiat.*, 5:569-612, 1965.

MEEKS, J. *The Fragile Alliance.* Baltimore: Williams and Wilkins Co., 1971, pp. 48-87.

NICHOLI, A. The adolescent. In Armand M. Nicholi, Jr. (Ed.), *The Harvard Guide to Modern Psychiatry.* Cambridge, Mass.: The Belknap Press of Harvard University Press, 1978.

OFFER, D. *The Psychological World of the Teenager.* New York: Basic Books, 1969.

RUTTER, M., LEBOVICI, S. ET AL. A tri-axial classification of mental disorders in childhood: An international study. *J. Child Psychol. Psychiat.*, 10:41-61, 1969.

SODDY, K. *Clinical Child Psychiatry.* London: Balliere, Kendall, and Cox, 1960.

SPITZER, R. & SHEEHY, M. D.S.M. III: A classification system in development. *Psychiatric Annals*, 6(9):102-109, 1976.

STRAUSS, J. S. The comprehensive approach to psychiatric diagnosis. *American Journal of Psychiatry*, 132(11):1193, 1975.

THOMÄ, H. Beobachtung und Beurteilung von Kindern und Jugendlichen. *Psychologische Praxis*, 15:1-64. Basel, 1953.

WERKMAN, S. The psychiatric diagnostic interview with children. *Amer. J. Orthopsychiat.*, 35:764, 1965.

WESTLEY, W. & EPSTEIN, N. *The Silent Majority.* San Francisco: Jossey-Bass, 1969.

6

Psychological Testing of Adolescents

REBECCA E. RIEGER, PH.D.

Psychological testing can contribute to the evaluation and treatment of adolescents in multiple ways. Within the larger framework of a full psychiatric evaluation, which typically includes history-taking with the parents and a diagnostic interview with the adolescent, at the minimum, psychological testing can offer an organized, systematic evaluation of the adolescent's functioning in the intellectual area, in the emotional sphere, and in the area of interpersonal perceptions and attitudes. It can describe the defensive system, fantasy investment, and self-concept. And it can speak to the mode, the level, and the success of adaptation to reality demands, as well as the degree of strain experienced in the adaptive process. Not all psychological testing with all adolescents will yield so broad a range of information, but the potential for gathering and evaluating such information is inherent in the diagnostic testing process.

RELATIONSHIP TO OVERALL ASSESSMENT

The place of the psychological examination in the temporal sequence of the full diagnostic study may vary. The testing may be used as a preliminary screening to identify problem areas for further exploration in the psychiatric interview or history-taking. For example, the test findings may suggest focal concerns over sexual identity or severe sibling rivalry, or anxiety over long deferred confrontation of being an adopted child, pointing the way to further

101

exploration. More traditionally, the psychological examination follows one or more psychiatric interviews and history-taking sessions, and may be used to investigate hypotheses derived from these interviews. For example, there may be a suspicion of a thought disorder, or a constitutional chronic learning problem, or concern over possible sociopathic trends; testing could, then, be focused specifically upon these issues.

In treatment planning, the psychological examination may be used to evaluate ego strength, coping ability, covert assets, and suitability for various treatment modalities, such as individual dynamically oriented psychotherapy, activity group, intensive psychoanalytic treatment or behavior modification, and could help make the decision regarding outpatient, residential or inpatient hospital treatment.

The psychological examination may also contribute to the evaluation of change associated with psychotherapy, other kinds of treatment (such as residential treatment experience) or environmental manipulation such as a change of school. It offers (from a somewhat more "objective" vantage point) a systematic "structural" view of change as reflected in cognitive functioning, defensive style, developmental level, affective reactivity, interpersonal perceptions, ego strength, and above all, self-concept.

Often, before change is perceptible in relation to coping in the real world, it is adumbrated in test behavior and response. To illustrate this point, consider the case of a 13-year-old "underachiever" in school: Testing revealed an adolescent of above average intelligence whose feelings of inadequacy and impotence were apparent in both the verbal and nonverbal spheres. To the question "What should you do if you saw a train approaching a broken track?" he said, "I know that I could signal, but what's the use—the engineer would look down the track, see a little kid, and ignore him!" Asked to draw a person, he produced a primitive ovoid body with spindly legs, a large head, and no arms. After a year in treatment, he was retested at the request of the psychiatrist, who saw little evidence of change. On the second occasion, his answer to the "train approaching a broken track" question was a crisp "Signal it," and his figure drawing showed very skinny, lightly sketched arms attached to an essentially unchanged body. The inference drawn from these (and other test findings), that he was beginning to feel less helpless, and that behavioral changes were likely to follow, proved correct. His grades started climbing steadily and he began to assume a more active role socially.

ASSUMPTIONS OF TESTING

The usefulness of test data rests on the basic assumption that in eliciting responses to a wide range of stimuli, in an interview-like, two-person situation, the psychologist can draw inferences and translate the findings into conclusions about behavior in the real world. A similar assumption applies equally to the psychiatric interview. Testing is also predicated on eliciting a representative sample of behavior, broad enough to encompass basic cognitive, affective, temperamental and motility aspects of personality functioning. Thus, it demands a battery of tests, rather than single instruments, however complex and "powerful" (e.g., the Rorschach). It demands a group of tests designed to sample nonverbal as well as verbal responses, covert as well as overt processes, and unconscious and/or suppressed as well as conscious and accessible content.

Throughout, there is a developmental focus which keeps in mind the normal succession of stages of maturation psychosexually, socially, cognitively and physically. Testing may, therefore, highlight whether the adolescent shows successful mastery of the stage-appropriate tasks. The adolescent is compared with his peer group, according to available norms—either developed in the course of standardization of tests like the intelligence scales, or developed empirically in the course of extensive experience over time (for tests such as the Rorschach and Bender Visual Motor Gestalt Test). The adolescent can also be described in terms of his stage of development, such as in the Piaget approach to cognitive maturation, which posits an orderly progression of stages and permits a judgment about the actual level of intellectual maturity, not only relative standing in the peer group: Has the adolescent passed from the stage of "concrete operations" into the stage of "formal operations"?

Along these lines, the psychological examination can contribute to the investigation of the "autonomous ego functions" and their direct derivatives—that is, developmental maturation aspects of psychobiological growth—such fundamentals as memory, perception, motility, stimulus barrier and affect-expression; and the derivatives, cognitive development, language development, concept formation, and synthetic functions of the ego.

Unlike a "talking" interview with an adolescent, the tests provide an opportunity to observe motility patterns, level of maturation of the perceptual-motor apparatus, the basic level of stimulability and impulse control, and reactions to task-related stress (as opposed to interpersonal stress, which could be explored very adequately in an interview). Task-related stress may be invoked in essentially neutral tasks which involve school-related questions, or visual-motor exercises, or work demanding close attention and concentration (such as the Coding on the WISC and equivalent Digit Symbol on the WAIS). Responses to such tasks within the psychological tests can give information about conflict-free areas of functioning, the efficiency of central nervous system processing, impulse control, and coping "style," including defensive structure.

Test results can help to sort out present maladaptive functioning from higher potential functioning and give some indication of the contingencies under which various behaviors are likely to be elicited, i.e. from a study and comparison of results on the different types of tests, and from intra- and inter-test variability, as well as from behavior during the test, including relationship to the examiner. Results can be expressed in terms of probabilities, such as "under certain specified conditions, it is likely or unlikely that the adolescent will respond in a certain way." As an example, an adolescent with strong impulses, very poor capacity for self-organization and self-regulation, as revealed in high scores on a structured intelligence test but serious difficulty with the ambiguity of the Rorschach, would be more likely to succeed in a structured classroom and school setting than in an open classroom with permissive standards and minimal adult supervision.

THE ADOLESCENT AND THE EXAMINER

In testing adolescents, the examiner's principal problem is probably the adolescent's perception of the examiner as an agent of the parents, school, psychiatrist, court, or other authority institution. Developmental issues also color the response to testing—issues of basic trust, autonomy and establishing competence. The examiner is almost always initially viewed with suspicion and/or anxiety. However, with very rare exceptions (cases of intractible suspicion and hostility which often represent serious pathology in the establishment of basic trust), a supportive, empathic, but minimally intrusive examiner can form a brief working alliance with the adolescent, enabling cooperation in the testing. It is helpful if the adolescent can be led to see the examiner as his or her agent, to ask and get an answer to the implied question: "What's in it for *me*?"

SPECIAL INDICATIONS FOR TESTING

From the broad spectrum of adolescent problems, certain types of problems are most in need of input from the psychological examination.

1) *Depression.* Where behavior has been dangerous and/or self-destructive or where significant depression is suspected, testing is needed, particularly if the adolescent is non-communicative and appears to be withholding information about affect, fantasy and plans. The test findings, because they involve interpretation at a symbolic level or where stimuli elicit unconscious material, may give information despite the conscious desire of the subject to hide sensitive data. For instance, there are "suicide indicators" in the Rorschach, derived from the protocols of completed and attempted suicides, which are not primarily in the realm of content and therefore not under the conscious control of an unsophisticated subject.

2) *Academic Problems.* Where there has been a history of school problems, with or without confirmed learning disabilities, the psychological examination can help put in perspective the role of academic failure in the current difficulties, e.g., depression as a primary response to long-standing school difficulties versus school problems secondary to emotional disturbance. There is a frequent phenomenon of depression in learning-disabled adolescents when the chronic learning disability fails to disappear after years of remedial efforts. It is important to assess the current status of the "structural" disability, to determine whether it is still active, partially compensated for, or essentially overcome.

3) *Neurological Disorders.* Psychological testing is advisable where deviant behavior is suspected of having associated neurological dysfunction, e.g., alterations in states of consciousness, as in the epilepsies; distortion in language usage, as in the aphasias; memory deficits; and seemingly unmotivated emotional outbursts.

4) *Treatment Planning.* Finally, psychological evaluation is suggested where differential diagnosis is important, with possible consequences for mode and locus of treatment, including indications for medication, and issues of hospitalization vs. residential treatment vs. day treatment vs. outpatient status. Included here is the question of suitability for intensive analytic therapy, especially in consideration of the heavy investment of time and financial resources for the family.

BASIC TEST BATTERY FOR ADOLESCENTS

The professional referring a patient for a psychological evaluation should communicate the reason for the referral as clearly and forthrightly as possible. The evaluation may go beyond a specific referral question when the examiner feels that other data are available and pertinent which may cast light on the presenting problem. It is inadvisable to make a referral that is instrument-centered, such as the request that the adolescent be given "just projectives" or, even more specifically, "the Rorschach." The choice of instruments is best left to the psychologist to answer the referral questions most adequately. A basic battery of tests for an adolescent migh include the following tests.

1) An intelligence test, such as the WISC-R, WAIS or Stanford-Binet. These are multidimensional tests, made up of diverse tasks, verbal and nonverbal, and therefore excellent clinical instruments to observe behavior, competence and coping strategies. They can also yield information about an adolescent in relation to his peers (or where the test has not been standardized to include minority groups, it may yield information about the adolescent's ability to compete in the majority society. Tests are increasingly standardized to include minority subjects) .

2) The Bender Visual Motor Gestalt Test, a totally nonverbal,

non-language test, involving the copying of designs. It can yield information about basic perceptual-motor maturity, management of motility, impulse press and impulse control. It can also reveal basic temperamental characteristics such as attitudes toward self-organization and orderliness. For example, a late adolescent patient, who was hospitalized after about two years of dangerous acting-out involving serious drug abuse and sexual promiscuity, was tested while an inpatient. In appearance and in behavior she presented herself as an unkempt, oppositional, scattered young woman. Her test responses were generally disorganized, sometimes negativistic, and at times floridly bizarre, particularly on the Rorschach (where she was reporting LSD flashback images). However, her Bender was executed with precision, well spaced, orderly, and in sharp contrast to the other tests. After the formal testing session, the examiner asked her help in understanding the glaring inconsistency. She laughed, and pointing at the Bender, said, "Until I was 16, *that* was the way I was!" Her massive adolescent rebellion had followed the divorce of her parents and the dissolution of the family home. A favorable prognosis, based largely on the Bender findings, proved to be accurate—she utilized treatment very well and left the hospital showing substantial improvement.

3) Human Figure Drawings (or House-Tree-Person) yield information about self-concept and internalized body image. For the adolescent, it gives information about attitudes toward sexual maturation and acceptance of a sexual role.

4) The Most Unpleasant Concept is an interview technique in which the adolescent is asked to draw "the most unpleasant thing you can think of," from which it is possible to gain insight into the critical conflict, affect and fears. To illustrate the range of answers, one adolescent girl drew a girl's bedroom, with a man entering the room through a window, whereas another drew a little spider. One adolescent boy (with growing paranoid symptomatology) drew a tiny figure on a high platform, surrounded by many other figures staring at him, whereas another boy drew a little baby drowning in a bathtub. The theme of violence is frequent, expressed in the "atom bomb" or in the drawing of a single gun.

5) The Rorschach is an associational, perceptual task, defined by

Herman Rorschach as "a diagnostic test based on perception." It is particularly distinguished by the degree of ambiguity and lack of structure inherent in the task, in contrast to tests like the intelligence scales, the Bender, and even the figure drawings. From the Rorschach can be determined locus of anxiety, stimulus barrier, affective reactivity, fantasy, defensive structure, interpersonal perceptions, and adequacy of reality testing. It also yields information about the self-concept.

6) The Thematic Apperception Test (T.A.T.) (or other "content" test, such as the Make-A-Picture-Story or a sentence completion) yields information on interpersonal perceptions of a conscious or preconscious nature, in more direct relation to the family and social environment, as well as indications of the individual's social role, needs, environmental pressures, and mode of conflict resolution.

7) Where school achievement tests results are not available, the adolescent's academic competence and achievement level can be gauged from the Wide Range Achievement Test and the Peabody Individual Achievement Test, among many others testing reading, spelling, computation and language arts.

There are many self-administered questionnaires to tap attitudes, interests, vocational preferences, and diagnosis. The most widely used is the Minnesota Multiphasic Personality Inventory (M.M.P.I.), a questionnaire which establishes a diagnostic category and behavioral potential by comparing the test profile to profiles of known diagnostic groups. There exist adolescent norms, making it a useful tool for those who are not primarily interested in the dynamic integration of multiple aspects of personality functioning in a unique adolescent.

There are also more specialized tests, or test batteries, to pursue the investigation of hypotheses derived from the basic battery: The Graham-Kendall Memory for Designs (for neurological impairment), the Wechsler Memory Scale (for evaluation of memory deficits), and the Reitan neuropsychological battery (to explore the dimensions of central nervous system dysfunction as to locus, chronicity, nature of pathological process, and even prognosis); this battery is best invoked after there is some preliminary investigation of possible neurological factors.

THE INTERPRETATIVE INTERVIEW

The final step in the psychological evaluation is the communication of the results and recommendations to the referral source, who may be a psychiatrist, another mental health professional, a pediatrician, the school, or the parents themselves. Where the referral comes from another professional, the psychologist may or may not be directly involved in the interpretation to the family and to the adolescent. Where the referring professional anticipates resistance to recommendations, it is useful to have a joint interpretive session, or to follow up the overall interpretation with a meeting with the psychologist to discuss the test findings more fully.

Where there are significant data referring to learning problems, it is advisable for the psychologist to be personally involved in the interpretation to the adolescent and family, and to the school, at the request of the parents, since the psychologist will be the most competent to discuss educational/remedial issues.

In any case, the results of the psychological evaluation must be integrated with the developmental and social history and information about current functioning in order to strengthen the relevance of the findings and the recommendations.

REFERENCES

AMES, L. B., MÉTRAUX, R. W., & WALKER, R. N. *Adolescent Rorschach Responses, Revised Edition.* New York: Brunner/Mazel, 1971.

HIRSCH, ERNEST A. *The Troubled Adolescent As He Emerges on Psychological Tests.* New York: International Universities Press, 1970.

LEVITT, EUGENE E. & TRUUMAA, AARE. *The Rorschach Technique with Children and Adolescents; Application and Norms.* New York: Grune & Stratton, 1972.

LOURIE, R. S. & RIEGER, R. E. Psychiatric and psychological examination of children. *The American Handbook of Psychiatry,* Second Ed., 2:3-36, 1974.

SCHILDKRAUT, M. S., SHENKER, I. R., & SONNENBLICK, M. *Human Figure Drawings in Adolescence.* New York: Brunner/Mazel, 1972.

7

The Diagnostic Spectrum in Adolescent Psychiatry: DSM II and DSM III

JUDITH L. RAPOPORT, M.D.
and
RACHEL GITTELMAN, PH.D.

The focus of this chapter is on the concept of a "good diagnosis" and on the changes between the American Psychiatric Association's *Diagnostic and Statistical Manual III* (forthcoming sometime in 1979), and its predecessor, *DSM II;* special reference will also be made to particular diagnostic issues in adolescent psychiatry, as they have been reflected in *DSM III.* The first section of this chapter borrows heavily from "Diagnostic Classification and Pharmacological Indications" (Gittelman-Klein, Spitzer and Cantwell, 1978), which the interested reader should read for greater detail on *DSM III* and the *International Classification of Disease (ICD) 9.*

CONCEPT OF DIAGNOSTIC PROCESS

A diagnosis should communicate the phenomenology of the disorder, i.e., the clinical symptoms grouped under the common label. Doing so provides a consensus which enhances the communicative value of diagnostic terms. However, a diagnosis should do more than indicate a clinical picture.

Ideally, a diagnosis has several characteristics. It should provide a good estimate of the natural history of the disorder (outcome or prognosis without treatment), its outcome given current treatment, its etiologies, the pathophysiology of the disorder if there is a specific biological cause, and, if there is a psychosocial cause, the psychological mechanisms underlying the disorder. These prognostic and etiological data are those necessary in the end to validate the syndrome and show that it is more than an arbitrary group of signs and symptoms. When all these factors are known, the ground is laid out not only for curing the disorders, but, better yet, for preventing them. Of course, the process of discovery does not usually proceed in this orderly fashion and the establishment of specific treatments may help to define clinical syndromes, such as might prove to be the case with depression or hyperkinetic disorder.

Unfortunately, very few psychiatric disorders of children or adolescents have been investigated sufficiently so that it may be stated with confidence that they have the associated etiological, prognostic, therapeutic and preventive validating factors discussed above. Though this uncertainty is unfortunate, it should act to stimulate systematic research in diagnosis in child psychiatry rather than lead to a defeatist attitude. There is certainly room for significant improvement in current diagnostic practice, but the usefulness of diagnoses also rests on the ability of the symptoms to reflect discrete clinical categories meaningful for interventions. There may be, for example, a better chance of finding the right drug after having identified the right diagnosis through an improved taxonomy. An obvious example of the value of a good taxonomy is the use of lithium in manic-depressive disorders. The syndrome was identified long before the use of the drug and thus facilitated the discovery of lithium treatment in those disorders. It is hoped that the improvements in the current diagnostic system for children (which most are agreed is unsatisfactory) may set the stage for the discovery of relationships between specific disorders and specific treatments (not necessarily pharmacological).

There are alternative concepts in diagnosis; behavioral scientists often use a dimensional approach in which behaviors are conceived of as dimensions like height or weight. In such a scheme, abnormality will be simply an extreme position. However, while such an approach has been used a great deal in research, it is at variance with the medical model in which a diagnosis is considered either present or absent. In *DSM III*, specific criteria for a diagnosis are given which may involve specific features in the history, such as duration of symptoms, or presence or absence of other difficulties. This latter approach, that of the "medical model," is basically that of *DSM III*.

TABLE 1

DSM II and *III* Classifications for Disorders Usually Arising
in Childhood or Adolescence

DSM II (Taken from all categories where there is mention of childhood)	*DSM III* (as of March, 1978)

Mental Retardation
- 310 Borderline
- 311 Mild
- 312 Moderate
- 313 Severe
- 314 Profound
- 315 Unspecified

Special Symptoms
- 306.00 Speech disturbance
- 306.10 Specific learning disturbance
- 306.20 Tic
- 306.30 Other psychomotor disorders
- 306.40 Disorders of sleep
- 306.50 Feeding disturbance
- 306.60 Enuresis
- 306.70 Encopresis
- 306.90 Other special symptoms

Transient Situational Disturbances
- 307.00 Adjustment reaction of infancy
- 307.10 Adjustment reaction of childhood
- 307.20 Adjustment reaction of adolescence

Behavior Disorders of Childhood and Adolescence
- 308.00 Hyperkinetic reaction
- 308.10 Withdrawing reaction
- 308.20 Overanxious reaction
- **308.30 Runaway reaction**
- 308.40 Unsocialized aggressive reaction
- 308.50 Group delinquent reaction
- 308.90 Other reaction

Schizophrenia
- 295.80 Childhood

Mental Retardation
- 317.0 Mild
- 318.0 Moderate
- 318.1 Severe
- 318.2 Profound
- 319.0 Unspecified

Pervasive Developmental Disorders
- 299.00 Infantile autism
- 299.80 Early childhood psychosis
- 299.20 Pervasive developmental disorder of childhood, residual state
- 299.90 Unspecified

Specific Developmental Disorders
Note: These are coded on Axis II
- 307.6 Enuresis
- 307.7 Encopresis
- 315.00 Specific reading disorder, Alexia, Developmental Dyslexia
- 315.10 Specific arithmetical disorder
- 315.30 Developmental language disorder
- 315.40 Developmental articulation disorder
- 315.50 Coordination disorder
- 315.60 Mixed
- 315.80 Other
- 315.90 Unspecified

Stereotyped Movement Disorders
- 307.21 Motor tic disorder
- 307.22 Gilles de la Tourette
- 307.29 Unspecified tic disorder
- 307.30 Other

Speech Disorders Not Elsewhere Classified
- 307.00 Stuttering

Conduct Disorders
- 312.0 Undersocialized conduct disorder, aggressive type
- 312.1 Undersocialized conduct disorder, unaggressive type
- 312.2 Socialized conduct disorder

TABLE 1 (*continued*)

Eating Disorders
307.10 Anorexia nervosa
307.51 Bulimia
307.52 Pica
307.53 Rumination
307.58 Other or unspecified

Anxiety Disorders
309.21 Separation anxiety disorder
313.20 Shyness disorder
313.00 Overanxious disorder

Disorders of Late Adolescence
309.22 Emancipation disorder of
adolescence or early adult life
309.23 Specific academic or work
inhibition
313.60 Identity disorder

*Other Disorders of Childhood or
Adolescence*
313.xx Introverted disorder of childhood
313.50 Oppositional disorder
313.70 Academic underachievement
disorder
313.23 Elective mutism

*Other Disorders Commonly Diagnosed in
Childhood, But Not So Designated in
DSM III*
Sleep Disorders
307.46 Somnambulism
307.47 Night terrors

Psychosexual Disorders
302.61 Gender identity or role disorder
of childhood

Adjustment Disorders
300.40 with depressed mood
309.24 with mixed emotional features
309.28 with anxious mood
309.30 with disturbance of conduct
309.40 with mixed disturbance of
emotions and conduct
309.82 with physical symptoms
309.83 with withdrawal
309.90 other or unspecified

Differences Between DSM II *and* DSM III

There are considerable changes between *DSM III* and its predecessor, *DSM II*. There is a most striking increase in attention to disorders of childhood and adolescence, with about twice as many separate categories for disorders either exclusively or primarily used in childhood and adolescence in the new system.

Table 1 presents a comparison between *DSM II* and the proposed *DSM III* for Disorders Usually Arising in Childhood or Adolescence, and to which we have added some disorders not designated for childhood alone but which will be used frequently by child psychiatrists. Of course, children may receive diagnoses from the adult categories and that issue will be addressed later in this chapter.

There are also some general differences between *DSM II* and *III* which affect children. One change which is most noticeable is that the terms psychosis and neurosis are no longer used as grouping concepts. In addition to the many different uses of psychosis with adult patients (e.g., psychotic depression, psychotomimetic drug effects), there are particular difficulties with children. For example, children with autism are developmentally deviant from infancy on, and are frequently intellectually retarded. Therefore, for this group, the connotations which the diagnosis of psychosis carries are misleading.

"Neurosis" was abandoned because the term carries etiological inferences. As etiological speculations are not part of the new descriptive diagnostic terms, this category was abandoned.

All of the *DSM III* diagnostic descriptions will contain the following: 1) primary clinical features, 2) frequently but inconsistently associated secondary symptoms, 3) age at onset, 4) course of the disorder, 5) complications, 6) predisposing factors, 7) familial patterns, 8) prevalence, 9) sex ratio, 10) differential diagnosis, and 11) operational criteria for making the diagnosis. These descriptions represent a new attempt at description not in *DSM II*.

However, the most innovative idea for *DSM III* is the concept of the multiaxial approach. For this important change, child psychiatry can take a generous portion of the credit; some of those who worked on *ICD 9* (Rutter, Shaffer and Sturge, 1975) initiated this concept for children and it will now be applied both to children and adults. The point of this proposed change is to avoid the arbitrary basis on which diagnoses are sometimes made by symptom pattern (i.e., school phobia) or intelligence (i.e., mental retardation) or presumed etiology (i.e., adjustment reaction). It had been demonstrated that when children presented with a mixed clinical picture, categorization was inconsistent, as some diagnosticians would give weight to one aspect of a case (such as the presence of epilepsy in a child with conduct disorder) while others would focus on other aspects (such as IQ or situational stress).

In the proposed system, Axis I reflects the clinical disorder and it must be stressed that multiple diagnoses may be used. Axis II is for ratings of Specific Developmental Disorders (also in Table 1). These are deficiencies in development which cannot be accounted for by mental retardation or by deprivation. Axis II, therefore, will contain entities such as Specific Reading Disorder or Enuresis. While these disturbances have been shown to have a significant association with behavioral disturbance, they can, and often do, occur as isolated symptoms. In such cases, a child receives a diagnosis on Axis II alone.

Axes III, IV, and V of the proposed classification will not be covered here. In *DSM III*, Axis III will represent concurrent physical or biological disorders which are felt to be pertinent to the condition. For example, the presence of diabetes or asthma would be coded here, and could be of obvious relevance to the understanding of an adolescent psychiatric disorder.

Axis IV would provide information about psychosocial stress. This axis is still being developed; considerable thought has been given to the different stresses which are appropriate at different times of development. This category is to be used when a relationship between the disorder and the stress is inferred.

Axis V will note the highest level of previous functioning.

NEW DIAGNOSTIC CATEGORIES

As can be seen from Table 1, there is a greatly expanded list of diagnoses which will be used regularly for children and adolescents. In addition, there are over 100 diagnoses that also may be used for children; for example, it is expected that Sleep Disorders,

Reactive Disorders, and Psychosexual Disorders (which typically have onset during childhood) will be used regularly for children and adolescents.

The large number of disorders will seem bewildering and Kraepelinian to many practitioners. It is hoped that research technology of epidemiology, genetics, outcome, and response to different treatments will validate some and permit others to be discarded or combined.

DIAGNOSIS IN ADOLESCENT PSYCHIATRY

Regarding diagnosis in adolescent psychiatry, there are specific questions which should be considered: Are there diagnoses of adult disorders which are being overused or used inappropriately, or not sufficiently? Are there disorders specific to adolescence, or at least clinical patterns which have unclear relation to childhood or adult disorders so that they should be described separately?

The discussions surrounding these issues during *DSM III* Task Force Advisory meetings (Committee on Childhood and Adolescence*) were particularly provocative. The debate during *DSM III* committee meetings recapitulated some recurring dilemmas in adolescent psychiatry. Do adolescent diagnoses need a "separate status" from that for children or adults? Certain types of disability in adulthood clearly have origins during childhood or adolescence; Robins and co-workers have shown, for example, that antisocial disturbance typically originates during early adolescence (Robins, 1966). Similarly, while crucial matters such as type of treatment and prediction of outcome are still important areas of research with adolescents diagnosed as schizophrenic, there has been relatively greater follow-up work done on psychosis in adolescence (Gossett, Lewis, Lewis and Phillips, 1973) than in other areas, and this work has consistently demonstrated continuity between adult and adolescent psychosis.

------

* Members of the Advisory Committee on Childhood and Adolescent Disorders to the Task Force on Nomenclature and Statistics are: Robert Spitzer, M.D., Chairman, Robert Arnstein, M.D., Dennis Cantwell, M.D., Stella Chess, M.D., Everett Dulit, M.D., Rachel Gittelman, Ph.D., Richard Jenkins, M.D., J. Gary May, M.D., Judith Rapoport, M.D., Richard Ward, M.D., and Paul Wender, M.D.

DISORDERS CHARACTERISTIC OF LATE ADOLESCENCE

The area of greatest change, therefore, was in the addition of some new diagnostic labels in the relatively grey area of follow-up of late adolescent conditions seen often by college psychiatrists. A major portion of the work on this section was carried out by Robert Arnstein, M.D., from Yale University Student Health Service.

Three new diagnosis entities are presented here in their current form (as of January, 1978), in full. They are: Emancipation Disorder of Adolescence, Identity Disorder, and Specific Academic or Work Inhibition Disorder. The feeling of the committee members representing adolescent psychiatry was that these entities were not clearly related to childhood precursors; further follow-up information was lacking that would lead us to consider these disorders as early manifestation of disorders of later life (such as depression or schizophrenia). These diagnoses represent a departure in that they recognize the possibility of a phase specific crisis in late adolescent development, which *may* not have any continuous relationship to other disorders.

309.22 Emancipation Disorder of Adolescence or Early Adult Life

Essential Features. The essential feature is symptomatic expression of a conflict over independence following the recent assumption of a status in which the adolescent or young adult is more independent of parental control or supervision. The situation is associated with the expectable events of growing up and separating psychologically from the family. The individual consciously regards the change as desirable but internally experiences a conflict over the increased independence. Symptomatic expression may include difficulty making independent decisions commensurate with the new situation, increased dependence on parental advice, newly developed and unwarranted concern about parental possessiveness, adoption of values deliberately oppositional to parents, and rapid development of markedly dependent peer relationships. The diagnosis should not be made if the symptoms are secondary to any other mental disorder.

Associated Features. Erratic behavior in regard to independent actions may occur, including a kind of pseudo-independence. Eating and sleeping disturbances may occur, and somatic complaints may be voiced. Homesickness may be present if the individual has moved away from home. Depression and anxiety are frequently the most superficial features presented. Interference with study, if the individual is in an academic setting, or with work performance may also occur.

Age at Onset and Course. The age of onset is usually from 16 to 19, the age at which there is some expectation that individuals will become more independent from family. Symptoms suggesting this condition at later ages usually denote a more serious disorder. Common precipitating events are entrance into college, a full-time employment situation, or military service. The course is usually relatively brief; if it extends for more than a year, this usually suggests another disorder.

Impairment. Impairment generally is transient and mild, but rarely may be more severe.

Complications. Complications include possible interruption in school or employment progress.

Predisposing Factors. A history of parental ambivalence to independence on the part of the adolescent may be a predisposing factor.

Sex Ratio and Prevalence. Sex ratio and prevalence are not definitely known, although the condition can be observed in both males and females.

Familial Pattern. The familial pattern in not known.

Differential Diagnosis. Differentiation must be made from more serious disruptions of functioning, such as Schizophrenia Disorders or Affective Disorders. These are usually more severe and characterized by greater anxiety or mood disturbance. Separation Anxiety Disorder may appear to have some of the same features, but it is characterized by anxiety at separation and a wish to return to the parental home, whereas this disorder is characterized by a conscious desire for a situation involving independence from parental control and a concomitant conflict about such independence. In older adolescents the distinction may be less clear, but probably should be determined by whether the symptoms seem to stress problems relating to physical separation as opposed to psychological separation. Thus, homesickness as the major manifestation, because it emphasizes the physical separation, would suggest Separation Anxiety Disorder.

The condition must be distinguished from syndromes frequently seen in adolescents and young adults, such as Identiy Disorder and Adjustment Disorder. Identity Disorder involves a more fundamental concern with self-definition. Adjustment Disorder by definition also involves a reaction to an external situation or change, but it does not have the specific features of this disorder. The condition sometimes may need to be distinguished from Compulsive Personality Disorder in that difficulty in decision-making may be present in both, but this disorder lacks other characteristics of compulsivity. It must also be distinguished from Dependent Personality Disorder, which is usually more pervasive and represents a more ingrained pattern of pervasive character traits.

Table 2 summarizes the operational criteria for this new diagnostic category.

313.60 Identity Disorder

Essential Features. The essential feature is distress over an inability to reconcile aspects of the self into a relatively coherent and acceptable sense of self, not secondary to another mental disorder. The disturbance is manifested by intense subjective distress regard-

TABLE 2

Operational Criteria for Emancipation Disorder of Adolescence or Early Adult Life

A. Recent assumption of a situation in which the patient is more independent of parental control or supervision.
B. The patient regards the change as desirable.
C. Symptomatic expression of a conflict over independence is manifested by two or more of the following:
  1) Difficulty making independent decisions commensurate with a new situation.
  2) Increased dependence on parental advice.
  3) Newly developed and unwarranted concern about parental possessiveness.
  4) Adoption of values deliberately in opposition to parents.
  5) Rapid development of markedly dependent peer relationships.
  6 Homesickness which the individual finds inconsistent with a conscious wish to be away from home.
D. The condition is not secondary to any other mental disorder.

ing uncertainty about a variety of issues relating to identity, including long-term goals, career choice, friendship patterns, values, and loyalties. Frequently, this is summarized in the question, "Who am I?" The diagnosis is not made if the disturbance is symptomatic of another mental disorder such as Borderline or Affective Disorder.

The uncertainty regarding long-term goals may be expressed as inability to choose a life pattern—for example, one dedicated to material success or service to the community, or even some combination of the two. Conflict regarding career choice may be expressed as inability to decide or to pursue an apparently chosen field. Conflict regarding friendship patterns may manifest itself as attraction to particular groups who are characterized by opposite interests or styles. Conflict regarding values and loyalties may include concerns over religious identification, patterns of sexual behavior, and moral issues. The individual experiences these conflicts as irreconcilable aspects of his personality and as a result fails to perceive himself as having a coherent identity.

Associated Features. Frequently there is a marked discrepancy between the individual's view of himself and the view that others have of him. Mild anxiety and depression are common and usually related to inner preoccupation rather than external events. Self-doubt and doubt about the future are usually present, with either difficulty in making choices or impulsive experimentation. Negative or oppositional patterns are often chosen in an attempt to establish an independent identity distinct from family members or other close individuals. This may manifest itself as transient experimental phases of widely divergent behavior as the patient "tries on" various roles.

Age at Onset and Course. The most common age at onset is late adolescence or young adulthood as the individual becomes detached from his family value systems and attempts to establish his own identity. With changing value systems, this disorder may also appear later in life as individuals begin to question earlier life decisions. Frequently, there is an acute phase which either resolves over a period of time or becomes chronic. In other instances, the onset is more gradual. If the disorder begins in adolescence, it usually is resolved by the mid-twenties. If it becomes chronic, however, the individual may either be unable to establish career commitment or fail to form lasting emotional attachments, with resulting frequent shifts in jobs, relationships, and career directions.

Impairment. The degree of impairment varies but usually there is some interference with effective social functioning. Frequently, there is avoidance of goal-oriented tasks or a failure to complete them.

Complications. The most common complications are failure of educational achievement and work performance below that appropriate to intellectual ability.

Predisposing Factors. Inasmuch as the disorder has apparently become more common recently, predisposing factors may include a conflict between adolescent peer values and parental or societal values, and also reflect the greater number of options regarding values, behavior and life-styles open to the individual.

Sex Ratio, Prevalence and Familial Pattern. Unknown.

Differential Diagnosis. Identity Disorder should not be diagnosed if identity problems are secondary to another mental disorder. Differentiation from such conditions as Schizophrenic Disorders and Affective Disorders is self-evident. The diagnosis should not be made if there are marked disturbances in mood, thus warranting a diagnosis of Episodic Chronic, or Atypical Affective Disorder. Differentiation from Unstable Personality Disorder (Borderline Personality Disorder) may be difficult, but in the latter disorder identity conflict is only one of several areas of disturbance and there is often marked and sudden mood change. What appears initially to be Identity Disorder may later turn out to have been an early manifestation of Borderline Personality Disorder or Schizophrenic Disorder, but this can only be determined with time. Identity Disorder must also be differentiated from the ordinary conflicts associated with maturing; the latter are not associated with either severe distress or pervasive conflict. Individuals with Compulsive Personality Disorder may manifest identity problems and should be given both diagnoses if identity conflicts are prominent and not judged to be merely a manifestation of indecisiveness.

309.23 Specific Academic or Work Inhibition

Essential Features. The essential feature is a clinical picture dominated by a specific academic or work inhibition occurring in an

TABLE 3

Summarizes the operational criteria for Identity Disorder

A. Severe subjective distress regarding uncertainty about a variety of issues relating to identity, including long-term goals, career choice, friendship patterns, values, and loyalties.
B. Does not meet criteria for an Affective Disorder, Schizophrenic Disorder, Pervasive Developmental Disorder, or Unstable Personality Disorder (Borderline Personality Organization).
C. Age at onset not prior to 14.

individual whose intellectual capacity, skills, and previous academic or work performance have been at least adequate. The inhibition occurs despite apparent effort and is not due to any other mental disorder.

There is invariably severe distress with mixtures of anxiety and depression; this distress interferes significantly with some important academic or work activity. There may be anxiety over examinations; inability to write papers or reports or perform in studio arts activities; difficulty in concentrating on studies or work; or avoidance of studying or work which does not seem to be under the conscious control of the individual. The distress is not present when the individual is not thinking about the academic or work task.

Associated Features. In attempting to cope with anxiety and depression, individuals may develop insomnia and/or hypersomnia, rituals, and disorganization of daily routine. Sometimes the condition is accompanied by excessive alcohol intake or eating, increased drug use, or incessant smoking.

Age at Onset and Course. The onset may occur at any time during the course of an individual's academic or work life, but is more likely to occur in late adolescence. The course is highly variable. Improvement may occur gradually, or, if the disturbance is acute, the problem may resolve quickly and not recur. In some severe cases, it may be self-limiting because it leads to the termination of schooling which, in turn, eliminates the precipitating stress.

Impairment. Impairment is generally limited to academic consequences.

Complications. Interpersonal friction may develop with parents whose expectations are not met by the adolescent. If the symptoms occur in the college period, parents may be upset by the financial outlay which is being "wasted." Late adolescents and young adults may suffer possible interruption in academic work or in preparation for a selected career. If the disorder occurs in a work situation, the individual may suffer a job loss or demotion.

Predisposing Factors. Predisposing factors may include Compulsive Personality Disorder and a family environment that overly stresses achievement. The condition frequently occurs at the beginning of a new academic stage or at a critical moment leading to academic success, such as just prior to graduation or at the end of completion of a dissertation.

Sex Ratio and Prevalence. The disorder is relatively common and found equally in males and females.

Familial Pattern. There is no known familial pattern for the disorder.

Differential Diagnosis. This diagnosis is not given if the academic or work difficulties are caused by any of the Specific Developmental Disorders; the latter can be distinguished by specific tests. It may be distinguished from Academic Underachievement Disorder by the more specific nature of the difficulty and by the fact that the individual's distress is likely to be more acute. For all age groups the diagnosis should not be made if it is secondary to another mental disorder, such as Identity Disorder, Compulsive Personality Disorder, Depressive Disorder, or Anxiety Disorder.

DSM-III FIELD TRIALS

The format of these diagnoses represents that required for all of the diagnoses used in *DSM III.* It is hoped that the operational criteria will allow both epidemiological and follow-up information to be obtained. It was argued that these descriptions represent a significant advance in that they recognize that certain disorders may be transient and unique to a particular developmental phase. Nevertheless, considerable validating work will be required in order to ultimately justify the separate handling of these groups.

Field trials using these diagnoses have been carried out during 1976-77. Dr. Robert Arnstein was able to share the findings of the field trial from Yale Student Health Service (Arnstein, personal

TABLE 4

Summarizes the operational criteria for diagnosis of
Specific Academic or Work Inhibition

A. The predominant clinical feature is severe distress interfering significantly with
any of the following academic or work tasks and manifested by:
   1) Anxiety related to examinations or other tests.
   2) Inability to write papers or prepare reports, or perform in studio arts activities.
   3) Difficulty in concentration on studies or work.
   4) Avoidance of studying or work which does not seem to be under the conscious
   control of the individual.
B. Distress is not present when the individual is not thinking about the academic
work or task.
C. Adequate intellectual and academic or work skills.
D. Previous academic or work functioning has been at least adequate.
E. Intended academic or work effort even if secondarily extinguished by one of the
conditions included in A above.

communication). In his report, Arnstein found that the largest
single category was that of Adjustment Disorder, having a total
of 116 individuals (from 300 consecutive cases) being given one of
the subtypes. However, another large group consisted of patients
given the Late Adolescent Diagnoses which were developed specifically for this age group; 62 individuals were given these diagnoses. If students only were counted, 25% of these cases received
one of the three diagnoses described above in full (Emancipation
Disorder, Identity Disorder, or Work Inhibition Disorder).

The reactions of the clinic staff were in general favorable. The
Adjustment Disorder categories were felt to be more specific than
the prior Adjustment Disorder of Adolescence from *DSM II* while
avoiding the stigma or finality of Anxiety or Depressive Disorder.

The task force position on the new diagnoses of late adolescence,
however, seemed to us, by unofficial poll, rather conservative. Traditional views in adolescent psychiatry have held that there are often
transitory emotional crises which may blur the usefulness of diagnostic assessment. However, more recent work indicates that there is
really no justification for abandoning traditional psychiatric diagnosis for this age group (Masterson, Tucker and Berk, 1966; Masterson, 1967; Rutter et al., 1976; Weiner & Del Gaudio, 1976).
Whether these life disruptions of late adolescence will still be sepa-

rate disorders by *DSM IV* remains to be seen; several on the task force felt that they will be found to be early manifestations of adult disorders by subsequent validating studies.

A second concern surrounding diagnosis in adolescent psychiatry is something of the converse of the previous section. That is whether psychiatrists are missing diagnoses in adolescents which actually are clearly early manifestations of well-defined syndromes of adulthood. For example, until the recent activity of the Gilles de la Tourette Society and the interest in the use of haloperidol, that syndrome was frequently missed by child and adolescent psychiatrists only to be diagnosed later in life (Shapiro, Shapiro and Wayne, 1973).

In a recent study of Manic-Depressive Illness in Early Adolescence (Carlson and Strober, in press) the clinical phenomenology and course of illness were studied retrospectively for six cases who had the onset of bipolar manic-depressive illness in early adolescence. Despite original chart diagnoses of schizophrenia in *all cases,* systematic evaluation of clinic record data indicated that diagnostic manifestations of affective disorder were identifiable even at the onset of illness. The diagnosis was missed even though manic-depressive illness first becomes manifest between 10 and 19 years of age in one-third or more of bipolar affective patients (Winokur, Clayton and Reich, 1969; Perris, 1966). The advent of lithium treatment for such conditions makes these findings of more than academic significance.

A particularly interesting feature of the Carlson study was that closer examination of case records did *not* indicate that there was any obvious connection between typical adolescent phenomena and the content of clinical symptomatology. For example, concerns of vocation, academics, heterosexuality and independence from family were signs of recovery from the acute stages of the illness and not focal issues during the early phase. The data, therefore, did not support the notion that "adolescent turmoil" created a smoke screen around the true clinical picture.

In an important epidemiological and 10-year follow-up study of over 1,000 patients, Weiner and Del Gaudio (1976) have made a similar point with regard to the diagnosis of schizophrenia in adolescence. Their findings indicated that 14% of personality disorders and neurotics, 11% of those diagnosed as situational disorders and 20% of those diagnosed as "other" were subsequently considered to be schizophrenic. Their findings do not permit analysis of whether the clinical picture was truly obscure or whether the clinician was understandably hedging in making this diagnosis. With the demonstrated efficacy of phenothiazines in controlling some of the symptoms of psychosis, however, this finding is of more than academic interest. Future studies could profitably look at such cases in small, intense studies to see whether, as Carlson did for her bipolar group, earlier identification would have been possible. A useful study of this type is that of Ford, Hudgens and Welner (1978) in which 24 previously unclassified adolescents were followed up for seven years. At the conclusion of follow-up, 12 could be diagnosed by established syndromes; the presence of psychotic symptoms predicted outcome.

RELATED ISSUES IN CHILD PSYCHIATRY

We have focused on disorders in adolescence in relation to disorders in adulthood. We should look also at the diagnostic issues which adolescent psychiatry "inherits" from middle childhood phenomenology. Rutter has recently reviewed the question of diagnostic validity in child psychiatry in an excellent overview (Rutter, 1977). He finds good evidence for validation of some of the diagnostic distinctions that are commonly made. Infantile autism is a well-established condition, for example, which differs from other syndromes such as retardation and schizophrenia. Similarly, the general differentiation between conduct disorders and emotional disorders (neurotic disorders) also seems well-validated. However, there is still considerable debate over the entities of Childhood Depression and Minimal Brain Dysfunction for which Rutter believes diagnostic validity is not yet established.

With ongoing debates over the latter two categories, we would be on most shaky grounds to discuss the continuation of these syndromes into adolescence. We can speculate that the diagnosis of depression should be somewhat easier in adolescence where mood alteration may take a more recognizable form. On the other hand, Minimal Brain Dysfunction (renamed Attention Deficit Disorder in DSM III), is still the subject of considerable controversy. I would urge that any use of the Attention Deficit Disorder category for adolescents require a clear childhood history of restless inattentiveness and impulsivity during grade school years.

One should keep in mind the several provocative reports in recent years on Minimal Brain Dysfunction syndromes in young adults and adolescents. For example, Hartocollis (1968) described 15 inpatients at the Menninger Hospital who scored in the "middle range" for cerebral dysfunction; they were selected from patients between the ages of 15 and 25. These patients had received various diagnoses, including schizophrenic reaction, depressive reaction, and infantile personality. They had in common a history of behavior disorder since early childhood; many had minor congenital abnormalities suggestive of an underlying congenital disability of a general sort. Quitkin and Klein (1969) also described young adult inpatients in the same range as the Hartocollis sample. Those having suggestive signs of Minimal Brain Dysfunction (difficult birth history, childhood hyperkinesis, impulse disorder, clumsiness, learning problems or "organic" indicators on admission mental status) were examined for present symptom pattern. Two syndromes were described: a socially awkward withdrawn group lacking social skills; and an impulsive destructive group with social skills relatively intact. Finally, Cohen, Weiss and Minde (1972) described the persistence of the cognitive deficit of hyperactivity into adolescence as part of a follow-up study of childhood hyperactivity. Impulsive cognitive style and inattentiveness still characterized the adolescents in their sample. Still, delineation of an adolescent MBD syndrome seems premature; several current research efforts, however, are aimed at identifying adolescents and young adults with MBD who may also respond to stimulant medication. There will be a good deal in the forthcoming literature, therefore, about "adolescent hyperkinetics" (or "Adult MBD"), without clear consensus on how one should make the diagnosis in this age group (for which classroom teacher ratings are unavailable as there is usually no primary teacher); the muddle around this diagnosis will undoubtedly continue. Ratings by the patient, parents, and peer may prove useful but this remains a current research question.

Other questions arose with regard to the use of childhood disorders for older patients. For example, the diagnosis of "Separation

Anxiety," which is now a separate diagnosis under Childhood Conditions, was considered as a possible candidate for Emancipation Disorder described above. Arguments against this were, of course, that most Emancipation Disorder diagnoses were given to individuals who were not likely to have suffered from previous separation anxiety. This may or may not be the case, since one usually does not find such an association unless it is specifically sought. Diagnostic issues which also might be raised concern the adolescent manifestations of autism and other pervasive developmental disorders where, without the appropriate history, the current clinical picture can resemble other psychotic conditions, such as chronic undifferentiated schizophrenia.

RELATED ISSUES IN ADULT PSYCHIATRY

Finally, to return to the relation between adolescent diagnosis and that for the adult world, a thorny problem remains—as thorny for *DSM III* as it is for many of us in real life—how to handle the "couples" problem! There is a coding for Marital Problem and Other Interpersonal Problem under the section, "Conditions Not Attributable to Known Mental Disorder." There are no "dyadic" diagnoses, and some would argue that there should be special consideration to this issue during middle and late adolescence. This has not been addressed in *DSM III;* the hazards of romantic entanglements may be as unavoidable and uncontrollable for diagnostic nomenclature as they are in real life!

It is hoped that *DSM III* will be used with particular interest by practitioners as a form of clinical research. The diagnostic systems are only as good as the data on which they depend. Those working in the field of adolescent psychiatry are, therefore, urged to keep their own notes on their use of these categories, particularly the new Disorders of Late Adolescence. There are high hopes for the new diagnostic system—that it will permit greater clarity between centers and provide unique epidemiological data. The system will only be as good as the tolerance of the participating clinicians for completing the diagnostic coding system. It will be the level of participation, therefore, which will eventually determine the usefulness of *DSM III.*

REFERENCES

ARNSTEIN, R. Personal communication.

CARLSON, G. & STROBER, M. Manic-depressive illness in early adolescence. *J. Am. Acad. Child Psychiatry*, in press.

COHEN, N., WEISS, G., & MINDE, K. Cognitive styles in adolescents previously diagnosed as hyperactive. *J. Child Psychol. Psychiatry*, 13:203-209, 1972.

Diagnostic and Statistical Manual of Mental Disorders, II. Washington, D. C.: American Psychiatric Association, 1968.

FORD, K., HUDGENS, R., & WELNER, H.: Undiagnosed psychiatric illness in adolescents, a prospective study and seven year follow-up. *Arch. Gen. Psychiat.*, 35:279-288, 1978.

GAP Psychopathological Disorders in Childhood: Theoretical Considerations and a Proposed Classification. New York: Group for the Advancement of Psychiatry, 1966.

GITTELMAN-KLEIN, R., SPITZER, R., & CANTWELL, D. Diagnostic classification and psychopharmacological indications. In J. Werry (Ed.), *Pediatric Psychopharmacology— The Use of Behavior Modifying Drugs in Children.* New York: Brunner/Mazel, 1978.

GOSSETT, J., LEWIS, S., LEWIS, J., & PHILLIPS, V. Follow-up of adolescents treated in a psychiatric hospital. *Am. J. Orthopsychiatry*, 43:602-610, 1973.

HARTOCOLLIS, D. The syndrome of Minimal Brain Dysfunction in young adult patients. *Menninger Clinic Bulletin*, 32:102-114, 1968.

MASTERSON, J. F. *The Psychiatric Dilemma of Adolescence.* Boston: Little, Brown, 1967.

MASTERSON, J., TUCKER, K., & BERK, G. The symptomatic adolescent: Delineation of psychiatric syndromes. *Compr. Psychiatry*, 7:166-174, 1966.

PERRIS, C. A study of bipolar and unipolar recurrent depressive psychosis. *Acta Psychiatr. Scand.* (Suppl), 162:45-51, 1966.

QUITKIN, F. & KLEIN, D. F. Two behavioral syndromes in young adults related to possible Minimal Brain Dysfunction. *J. Psychiat. Res.*, 7:131-142, 1969.

ROBINS, L. *Deviant Children Grown-Up.* Baltimore, Maryland: Williams & Wilkins, 1966.

RUTTER, M. Diagnostic validity in child psychiatry. Paper presented at the Interdisciplinary Society of Biological Psychiatry, Amsterdam, October 14, 1977.

RUTTER, M., GRAHAM, P., CHADWICK, O., & YULE, W. Adolescent turmoil: Fact or fiction. *J. Child Psychol. Psychiatry*, 17:35-56, 1976.

RUTTER, M., SHAFFER, D., & SHEPHERD, M. An evaluation of the proposal for a multiaxial classification of child psychiatric disorders. *Psychol. Med.*, 3:244-250, 1973.

RUTTER, M., SHAFFER, D., & STURGE, C. *A Guide to a Multi-Axial Classification Scheme for Psychiatric Disorders in Childhood and Adolescence.* London: Frowde & Co., 1976.

RUTTER, M., SHAFFER, D., & STURGE, C. *A Multi-Axial Classification of Child Psychiatric Disorders.* Geneva: WHO, 1975.

SHAPIRO, A., SHAPIRO, E., & WAYNE, H. The symptomatology and diagnosis of Gilles de la Tourette Syndrome. *J. Am. Acad. Psychiatry*, 12:702-723, 1973.

WEINER, I. & DEL GAUDIO, A. Psychopathology in adolescence: An epidemiological study. *Arch. Gen. Psychiatry*, 33:187-193, 1976.

WENDER, P. *Minimal Brain Dysfunction in Children.* New York: Wiley, 1971.

WINOKUR, G., CLAYTON, P., & REICH, T.: *Manic-Depressive Illness.* St. Louis: C. V. Mosby, 1969.

Part III

TREATMENT

Part III reviews the indications, contraindications, and techniques of basic treatment modalities in adolescent psychiatry.

John E. Meeks introduces this section on treatment with a review of the concept of therapeutic alliance as it pertains uniquely to the adolescent patient. He reviews technical factors in achieving the alliance, and methods of avoiding some of the pitfalls which threaten the alliance during the course of therapy. Expanding on his earlier work, he also includes a discussion of the therapeutic alliance with severely disturbed adolescents.

Chapter 9, on *Individual Psychotherapy with Adolescents,* presents an overall developmental concept that can be useful in the selection of individual therapy. Kessler points out that neither a diagnostic label nor the severity of the symptom(s) is a clear indicator of a teenager's ability to utilize individual therapy. Case reports illustrate his concept.

Paul S. Weisberg reviews the indications and goals of group therapy. He also remarks comprehensively on the group leader, the composition of the group, frequency of meetings, role of the patient's family, and treatment termination.

In Chapter 11, *Adolescents in Family Therapy,* Roger L. Shapiro draws upon his research findings and describes the concept of complementary unconscious fantasies and related defenses within family members. He discusses the implications of his findings for the treatment of adolescents in family therapy and provides verbatim excerpts from family therapy sessions to illustrate his conclusions.

The subject of psychopharmacology in adolescent psychiatry is a "murky and uncharted field," according to the author of Chapter 12, Donald McKnew, Jr. The author recognizes well that adolescents require special scrutiny when psychotropic drugs are employed. Simply increasing the usual "child" dosage or decreasing the customary "adult" dosage is not enough. Dr. McKnew reviews the basic categories of psychotropic medications as to indications, dosage, and side effects.

Joseph R. Novello identifies the day hospital as a distinct, and underutilized, level of treatment in adolescent psychiatry. Four basic uses of the day hospital are described, along with programming outlines and staffing patterns. Selection of patients is stressed and outcome studies are reviewed.

The last chapter fittingly ends with the most intensive and most restrictive form of treatment in adolescent psychiatry: hospital treatment. William M. Lordi reviews the indications for hospitalizing an adolescent and describes programming criteria for intermediate-length hospitalization. Finally, he distinguishes between hospitalization and residential treatment for adolescents.

8

The Therapeutic Alliance in the Psychotherapy of Adolescents

JOHN E. MEEKS, M.D.

Approximately seven years ago the first printing of *The Fragile Alliance* (Meeks, 1971) appeared. It included an extended discussion of the nature of the therapeutic alliance in the psychotherapy of adolescents, the technical factors involved in achieving the alliance, and methods of avoiding some of the problems which threaten the alliance during the course of therapy. Since preparing that discussion, I have encountered very little that would negate the basic principles outlined there. Since the interested reader can review that extensive treatment of the issue, there seems little advantage in repeating the material included there in detail at this time. Instead, the basic principles described there will be reviewed only briefly here.

However, since writing that discussion, I have had the opportunity to interact extensively with large numbers of adolescents who would not, perhaps, fit all of the criteria for outpatient treatment described in *The Fragile Alliance*. Many of these adolescents were seen for therapy in an inpatient setting and were continued in outpatient treatment as part of their aftercare plans. Others were not treated as inpatients by the author but were referred for follow-up outpatient psychotherapy by other inpatient practitioners. These youngsters included a broad range of diagnostic categories, including schizophrenic adolescents, youngsters with borderline psychopathology, youngsters with severe disturbances in narcissistic development, and a variety of severe characterological disturbances.

Experiences with these young people have led gradually to a broadening of the concept of the therapeutic alliance. It has seemed evident that many of these adolescents are incapable of developing the degree of relatedness implied in the concept of the therapeutic alliance which is set forth in the *The Fragile Alliance*. However, in spite of this "deficiency" many of them show significant improvement in psychotherapy. Although there are many problems and questions which remain unanswered, some tentative observations and conclusions regarding the alliance in this sizeable group of adolescent patients will be offered following the brief review of previous material. Finally, some ideas regarding the formation and maintenance of a therapeutic alliance in inpatient treatment of the adolescent will be presented.

A BRIEF REVIEW OF THE THERAPEUTIC ALLIANCE IN OUTPATIENT PSYCHOTHERAPY OF ADOLESCENTS

I have previously stated that outpatient psychotherapy with adolescents should be undertaken only after some significant diagnostic questions are resolved in the course of a thorough evaluation.

1) *Is the adolescent genuinely concerned regarding some aspects of his psychological functioning?* As noted before, this can be a puzzling question in view of the adolescent's fear of appearing vulnerable or in need of a dependent relationship. It should not be expected that every treatable adolescent will voice openly and directly concern and desire for change. It is even less likely that the adolescent will anticipate that the therapy will be a safe source of assistance with any areas of difficulty that do concern him. The result is that many adolescents present with apparent denial of problems and rejection of help. However, the sensitive and alert practitioner can differentiate these anxious, face-saving maneuvers from a genuine acceptance of psychopathology with relative ease.

2) *Is the adolescent able to observe his own psychological functioning and report it with reasonable accuracy and honesty to the therapist?* Of course, there is no expectation that the adolescent will have the ability or the motivation to behave in this way during a diagnostic evaluation or the early phases of psychotherapy. However, tentative and tactful confrontations often make it evident that the young person has this capacity, as in the following case.

Case Report

A handsome, popular, 17-year-old young man was referred for psychotherapy because of psychosomatic problems. During the evaluation he emphasized his certainty that he had no emotional difficulties and his belief that psychiatric treatment was either quackery or, at best, a haven for losers and "weak-willed" people. When therapy was recommended and his parents required him to attend at least several planned exploratory sessions, he came to the first session but stated that he told his parents he would not come home that evening if they forced him to keep the appointment. The therapist asked about his motives in refusing to go home and he replied defensively that he was sure that the therapist thought he was "chickening out of a fight." The therapist stated that that idea had not occurred to him and that, in fact, he had been wondering if the decision was more of an effort to punish his parents since it seemed to the therapist that the patient actually was rather good at fighting and seemed to enjoy it. The patient grinned and said, "You are trying to say that I'm stubborn. If you had just asked I would have told you that. I'm about the most stubborn guy who ever lived."

3) *To what extent will the patient's family support therapy?* This question refers to the fact that individual psychotherapy is frequently quite threatening to parents. This is especially true when the adolescent's psychopathology is essential to the maintenance of a pathological family homeostasis. It also occurs in situations where the parents, for a variety of reasons, have difficulty in permitting the adolescent to form close attachments with anyone outside of the family boundaries. Regardless of the reasons, in families like this individual therapy is likely to be interrupted before its successful completion unless a prior course of family treatment or concomitant therapy of the parents is included in the treatment plan. In a very real sense one must have a therapeutic alliance with all significant family members, not just the designated patient.

ESTABLISHING ALLIANCE

The process of establishing a therapeutic alliance actually begins during the evaluation procedure. In a sense, deciding that a youngster is unhappy with some aspects of his personality, that he has the willingness and capacity to observe and describe himself, and that

his family has no vested interest in disrupting therapy—all actually
imply a beginning recognition of a developing alliance. Still, when
therapy begins officially, resistance often stiffens and the work of
establishing a firm therapeutic alliance begins in earnest.

I believe that the key to establishing a therapeutic alliance resides
in the careful and systematic interpretation of affective states as they
present early in the treatment process and particularly as they relate
to the interview situation itself. It is particularly important to be
alert to subtle distortions of the interpersonal relationship as it
develops in the here-and-now context of psychotherapy sessions.
These distortions may take many forms but represent conscious and
unconscious efforts by the adolescent to either negate the therapist
as a helpful person or to seduce the therapist into a neurotic interaction rather than a therapeutic one.

It might be useful to mention briefly some of the common forms
of early testing. The adolescent may invite the therapist to assume
an all-knowing and controlling position, may invite moral reproof
by threatening or implying antisocial behavior, or may challenge the
therapist to become competitive or to prove his therapeutic efficacy
immediately. As a rule, these maneuvers are relatively transparent
so long as one is comfortable with both the effectiveness and the
limitations of psychotherapy. If one can comfortably insist that the
only purpose of the sessions is to provide the patient and the therapist with a fuller understanding of the adolescent's true feelings,
it is relatively easy to understand and resist manipulations which
aim to distort the therapy process.

However, many psychological factors act to interfere with this
serene objectivity. One often encounters adolescent patients in an
atmosphere of crisis in which the therapist becomes the focus of
intense anxiety and concern emanating from parents, school officials,
referral sources, and other important adults in the community. The
pressure to "do something" about the chaotic situation can interfere
seriously with one's determination to approach the problem systematically and logically.

In addition, there may be some truth to the assertion that most
adults, even those who have undergone psychoanalysis, have re-
pressed the affects connected with their own adolescence. The result
is a spurious sense that one recalls and understands the personal

experience of the adolescent developmental period and its impact on adult functioning. Because of this defensive self-deception, we remain quite vulnerable to countertransference—motivated irrational responses to adolescent behavior. We can improve in this area only through experience, self-observation, and the regular use of supervision. Peer supervision seems particularly helpful in this instance since there is less tendency to defensiveness bred by reawakened adolescent conflicts in a supervisory process with an older or more experienced colleague. It is also extremely useful to review Keith's (1968) excellent paper on "unholy alliances." His clear exposition of the appearance of these untherapeutic relationships in child therapy is readily translated to adolescent work.

Although there are some objective evidences of the presence of the therapeutic alliance, a sucessful formation of the alliance is most readily recognized through a general tone of the therapeutic sessions. When an alliance exists, psychotherapy is characterized by a comfortable sense of mutual purpose but also carries a rather sobering overtone that the proceedings are serious and that matters of importance are at stake. Many therapists report that they experience a subjective sense of mild fatigue coupled with professional satisfaction on completion of a psychotherapy hour guided by a genuine therapeutic alliance.

It is also important to remember that the alliance is by no means static. The very work which is made possible by developing an alliance continually threatens the stability of the alliance as new defenses are recognized and challenged, new transference tendencies near consciousness, and areas of conflict and vulnerability are revealed to therapeutic scrutiny. At these times old or new resistances tend to characterize therapy sessions and the work of forming the alliance must be repeated before further genuine growth can occur in the therapy session. As a rule this is less difficult to accomplish than when first done at the time when therapy began because of the residual trust in the therapist's benevolence and steady insistence on a neutral inquiring attitude.

These comments should not be understood as a recommendation for a distant, unemotional, and totally cerebral approach to troubled adolescence. In fact, as Friedman (1969) has suggested in regard to the development of the therapeutic alliance in analytic work, formation of the alliance is probably possible only because of the patient's desire for a healthier experience of being nurtured. Friedman's paper points out that there is an inherent paradox in the notion that the patient's aim-inhibited, cooperative relationship with the therapist could be cemented by the very impulses which that relationship seeks to expose and modify.

These issues are even more marked in the adolescent patient, who tends to view most adults as either dangerous, potentially incestuous objects of the forbidden impulse life or, more frequently, as dessicated superego figures who oppose all pleasurable gratification. In fact, much of the early testing described above represents the adolescent's efforts to assure himself that he has found someone who will help him to grow in his own way and who will neither overstimulate his impulses to gain vicarious gratification nor oppose them because of neurotic inhibitions or generational envy. In short, the patient is looking for a parenting figure who will provide the opportunity for an internally harmonious maturation. It should be obvious that a therapist who appears cold, uncaring, and detached will hardly fit the patient's needs. However, the therapist who seems to have predetermined ideas regarding what is best for the patient or excessive needs to be liked by the patient or who appears excessively sympathetic or even overwhelmed by the young person's situation is equally unacceptable.

VARIATIONS IN THE PATTERN OF THE THERAPEUTIC ALLIANCE

In *The Fragile Alliance* I noted that when omnipotent transference tendencies in the adolescent were challenged "the adolescent usually reacts with irritation or open anger. This occurs because the transference actually covers the adolescent's secret fantasy of personal omnipotence. After all, the adolescent grants the therapist his power! It is also the adolescent who enjoys its benefits. The therapist serves as a dupe, fronting for the adolescent's defense against his fear of confronting reality without magical powers" (p. 127). In retrospect this is a naive and oversimplified view of the dynamics and structure of narcissistic transferences.

The work of Kohut (1971) and others has added a great deal to our understanding regarding the nature of narcissistic psychopathology and its expressions within the therapeutic relationship. Many adolescents with significant disturbances in narcissistic development need to aggrandize the therapist ("the idealizing transference") or to solicit endless admiration of themselves from the therapist ("the mirror transference"). In view of their desperate need to work through these developmental deficiencies within the therapeutic relationship it is small wonder that they react with anger if these patterns of relating are challenged or rejected. If the therapist is able to accept these feelings neutrally as any other distortion of his true nature and function would be accepted, the patient will gradually relinquish the unrealistic view.

Kohut has described the gradual disillusionment with the narcissistically invested idealized parental imago which characterizes normal development. This disillusionment occurs without any verbal disavowal of omnipotent perfection through the natural frustration of the patient's omnipotent hopes. In the author's experience, giving up this illusion is enormously painful and is often accompanied by alternating periods of depression and rage directed toward the therapist.

Case Report

Davy, a 16-year-old Caucasian male was admitted to a psychiatric hospital because of a suicide attempt. In the hospital setting he appeared markedly inhibited, frightened of his age mates, and often near psychotic in his fearfulness of the environment and his capacity to drift into long periods of reverie during which he seemed totally disinterested in his surroundings. The developmental history revealed that Davy had always been extraordinarily dependent on his mother, who regarded him as an extremely sensitive, intelligent, and "very special human being." He had never had good peer relationships and had tended to be the scapegoat in his classes throughout his school experience.

In his individual sessions Davy spoke very little to his therapist regarding personal matters. He was quite willing to discus his hobbies, which included sports (though he did not participate personally), literature, and music. In all of these areas Davy was extraordinarily well informed and showed a quick and incisive logic which was quite impressive for his age. When pressed to discuss his personal difficulties, including the suicide attempt, he would become evasive; if the pressure continued he would simply clam up.

However, in family therapy Davy began to express his concern about being overly dependent on his parents and began to ventilate feelings of frustration and anger when his mother's behavior seemed to him to be infantilizing. He also began to rebel against his scapegoated position in the peer group to the extent of becoming involved in physical fights on two occasions when he felt he was being "pushed around." As his general functioning improved, it was decided that Davy could be discharged from the hospital and followed in outpatient treatment. This decision was maintained in spite of the fact that Davy quickly reverted to his social isolation on his return home. Although he continued to verbally decry his inability to relate to people outside his family, he could not bring himself to make any active efforts to change that state of affairs.

In his individual treatment, Davy began to speak more freely about himself and his ideas. At the same time he seemed overly interested in the virtual "honor" of being a patient of his therapist. He was preoccupied with the therapist's national reputation, complimented the therapist on the brilliance and subtlety of his simplest statements and sang the therapist's praise to his family and anyone else who would listen. During this period he confided a variety of grandiose wishes and fantasies about himself and also recounted some embarrassing and frightening daydreams and wishes. He was particularly concerned regarding some homicidal fantasies and admitted that his suicide attempt was partially an effort to "rid the world of a potential murderer."

As the months went by, the unqualified admiration of the therapist continued but a new theme of identification with this power and Davy's self-adulation became more and more clear. For example, Davy would develop complex, imaginative metapsychological theory systems and present them in detail to the therapist. The manner of presentation suggested that Davy was attempting to earn the admiration of the therapist through emulation of the therapist's area of interest. Although there were some undercurrents of competitiveness, these seemed much less important than the desire to be praised by a "hero" figure.

Gradually, however, Davy began to look for clay feet. He devised situations, such as refusing to attend school, which created crises in which the therapist was powerless. He also showed a wry humor directed at the exalted image of the therapist which he had created. Usually, Davy reacted with open anger and disappointment when the therapist had to cancel appointments. During this period, however, Davy suddenly accepted an absence with cheerful indifference. When asked why he wasn't upset this time, Davy replied, "I've come to accept that it's just part of having a semi-famous psychiatrist."

Davy was quite depressed during this period. The disappointment of recognizing the therapist's human limitations and lack of magical power was clearly painful. Davy wavered between grief and rage toward the therapist. Only gradually was he able to begin to struggle realistically with his own life.

As Kernberg (1975) has noted, many of these youngsters utilize very primitive defenses, especially splitting. It is necessary while accepting the excessively positive transference to listen attentively to the feelings of rage and frustration expressed toward others since it can be assumed that these will eventually come into the transference also. In other cases, these youngsters may begin therapy with a primary demonstration of the negative side of their ambivalence. This is particularly likely because of projective identification which leads to fear that the therapist harbors those impulses and actions which are in fact struggling for expression in the youngster's own mind. Although the basic technical approach must include some interpretation of the fact that these are actually concerns and feelings of the patient, this must be done with some tact and skill to avoid a paranoid withdrawal from the treatment setting.

It is likely that we still have a great deal to learn about the skillful management of these youngsters who suffer severe impairment of early object relationships. However, it does seem clear that we must be open to a variety of therapeutic encounters which are quite different from the model of the therapeutic alliance as a relatively objective, cooperative expansion of the adolescent's observing ego.

Another variety of treatment relationship which seems constructive without actually measuring up to the traditional model of the alliance occurs with youngsters who have superego pathology. Johnson (1965), in her writings on the superego lacunae, described a major aspect of therapy related to the therapist's performance as a incorruptible model. Other authors have emphasized the same point (Meeks, 1978). For example, in treating youngsters with superego pathology the therapist must remain comfortably alert to the inevitability of efforts to corrupt his conscience. The patient will, with varying degrees of subtlety, attempt to corrupt the therapist into some minor bending of the rules which often appears harmless on the surface. When the therapist consistently accepts this maneuver good naturedly and without criticism but insists on "playing according to the rules," the patient frequently makes gains in superego development.

Other youngsters utilize the therapist in ways reminiscent of patterns described by Aichhorn (1935) to shore up their insufficient reality testing and superego controls. One 15-year-old youngster with a history of repeated juvenile offenses insisted that he "didn't give a damn" what the therapist thought of his activity. Still, when he was tempted to engage in antisocial activity, he would challenge the therapist to describe what he would do in the situation to avoid getting into trouble. Inevitably, the patient would scoff at the advice and then invariably would follow it. He would then return to the next session to complain that the solution did not work. In fact, the youngster showed continued growth and development, not only avoiding legal problems but showing steady improvement in schoolwork and family relationships.

Another violent 15-year-old boy with strong delinquent tendencies showed sudden and persistent improvement in his functioning in an inpatient adolescent unit. When asked by another youngster why he had stopped fighting with everyone, the patient explained, "My doctor is a champion boxer, I don't want to tangle with that guy." In fact, the therapist, was 10 pounds lighter than the patient and had not boxed in 20 years. In these instances, the patient creates the therapist in the kind of image that he requires to feel protected from his own tendencies to lose control. It is important to recognize that these fierce images of strict control are needed on an emergency basis and to quietly accept such projections. They can be gradually and helpfully modified by demonstrating in the direct management of the patient a warmer, less punishing, but still reliable style of impulse control.

Again, we are on relatively uncharted ground. The full implications of accepting alliances of this kind are difficult to evaluate fully. The problem, of course, is that these alliances are based on an unrealistic view of the therapist's actual personality and functioning and are not subject to honest appraisal and discussion. They must be viewed as temporary stages in treatment and, as Aichhorn said, it may be that the therapist who provides this help cannot continue the treatment when the patient is ready for a more intensive and dynamic treatment experience. In some cases, however, it does seem possible for the patient to understand the nature of the previous relationship and his past need for a distorted image of the therapist. In these cases it is possible to work through the previous style of relating and move toward a more traditional alliance.

One can approach these treatment relationships with the same questions which shed light on transference patterns with any patient. "How does the patient seem to wish to view me?" "What does he want from me?" "What is this doing for his psychological functioning?" When these questions are answered with some degree of accuracy, it permits the therapist to at least consider a further question: "To what extent is it ethical and comfortable for me to serve this function for the adolescent patient?" Giovacchini (1974) has described one type of patient who is extremely difficult to tolerate because his transference needs challenge the basic identity of the therapist as a helping person. His excellent article on "The Difficult Adolescent Patient" should be carefully reviewed. One final question must be asked: "Can this style of relating eventually lead to healthier psychological functioning for the adolescent patient?" It does seem possible to assist many adolescents without ever achieving a genuine therapeutic alliance. Perhaps. what happens in these cases is that the patient creates in the person of the therapist a particular adult image which can be internalized not as a transference object, but as a "real object" (Adatto, 1966), so that psychological maturation can continue.

THE THERAPEUTIC ALLIANCE IN THE INPATIENT
TREATMENT OF ADOLESCENTS

Some form of basic cooperation in the treatment effort is essential to success in the psychotherapy of any adolescent. This requires an agreement between the therapist and the patient (which may not be verbalized directly) that there is a psychological problem and that the adolescents will permit the therapist to assist in its solution. Many features of inpatient treatment obscure and complicate the development of this basic understanding even beyond its obfuscation in the outpatient treatment of the adolescent.

First of all, the adolescent is usually to some extent "confined" in the inpatient settting. In some instances the adolescent is at least verbally opposed to hospitalization and is in treatment only because the parents, the juvenile court, or other community agencies have forced his compliance. Even when the adolescent has been "voluntarily" admitted, he will usually protest his status as an inpatient at some point in treatment. If the therapist feels that inpatient treatment is necessary he is forced into a position of being the patient's "jailer" at the same time that he attempts to function as a therapist. Obviously this is fertile ground for the popular adolescent defense against autonomy: the projection of personal responsibility. It is easy for an adolescent who is being held in hospital treatment against his wishes to insist that any observed problems are the natural reaction to this abridgment of his civil rights. If this point is conceded, there is no therapeutic alliance, since the treatment is clearly the doctor's responsibility and the patient can choose only between passively complying with expectations so that he can go home or bravely and independently resisting the ominous and unfair control being exercised by an institution over a helpless individual.

This set of circumstances requires certain modification in the psychotherapeutic approach to the adolescent. Confrontation becomes more important, since the patient must be continually faced with the internal origin of his problems. Fortunately, accurate confrontation is much easier because of the wealth of information available from the 24-hour observation of the patient's behavior. With this data, it is often possible to convincingly demonstrate to the patient that he cannot handle the demands of life outside of the hospital setting until certain problems are resolved. It is very helpful in this process to obtain the support of the patient's peers in group settings. This is easier said than done. The subject of creating a pro-therapy atmosphere in inpatient adolescent units is beyond the scope of this paper. The detailed discussion presented by Lewis, Gossett, King and Carson (1970) remains a classic on the subject.

Another feature of inpatient psychotherapy which often startles and confounds therapists inexperienced in that type of work is the intensity of anger expressed by the patients. Often this is viewed as evidence of the more severe psychopathology present in the child who requires hospitalization. To some extent this is true but it does not account entirely for the phenomenon. In addition, there are the interacting factors of the safety of the structured inpatient setting and the "legitimate complaint" of having one's life rather completely monitored and controlled. At any rate, it is important to recognize that the presence of intense, regularly expressed anger in the treatment relationship does not suggest that the alliance is unworkable. To some extent the entire treatment process must be organized around a sometimes angry negotiation regarding the youngster's readiness for discharge (Meeks, 1968). It is also true that the therapist can afford a more open and firm expression of expectations regarding the level of behavior necessary for successful treatment to occur.

Case Report

An inpatient adolescent psychotherapy group was avoiding important and depressing treatment issues by clowning, interrupting one another, teasing the therapist and generally producing chaos. The therapist made several efforts to comment on the defensive nature of the behavior and to deal with the problems in a traditional psychotherapeutic way. These were totally ineffective. Finally, in exasperation the therapist shouted, "If I had wanted to teach nursery school I would have gotten training for that instead of learning to be a psychiatrist! You are all behaving like a bunch of little brats."

The group did not take offense. They laughed, said, "Wow, we've never seen you get mad," and proceeded to settle down and work on important issues.

Similar, although less flamboyant, candor is possible in individual sessions also. These liberties are possible because of the greater intimacy of the inpatient experience which makes it unlikely that patients will misunderstand the therapist's overall intentions toward them. Of course, there is also much greater support both from the many other staff members which the patient relates with and from the other members of the patient group.

Although the therapist should consistently confront the patient with his need for treatment and refuse to accept the assigned responsibility for the patient's welfare, it should also be recognized that most adolescents should not be expected to openly avow their need for treatment no matter how desperate that need may be. In fact, when patients speak too fluently of their need for treatment, seasoned inpatient practitioners become suspicious that such talk is a maneuver to gain earlier discharge through an appearance of "insight."

Severe Acting-Out

The implications for the treatment relationship of severe episodes of acting-out are sometimes difficult to understand. The variety of concurrent important relationships which are impinging on a young-ster in inpatient treatment sometimes stagger one's efforts to gain a clear picture of the relative importance of each. The patient's rela-tionship with his family, with significant nursing staff personnel, with other patients and with friends outside of the hospital must all be considered in trying to understand why a youngster has run away from the hospital, erupted into physical violence, brought drugs into the inpatient setting, or in some other way departed strikingly from treatment expectations. It is very possible that the relationship with the psychotherapist is often underestimated as a participant of these behaviors. Acting out is a common form of re-sistance in the adolescent in outpatient psychotherapy. It becomes a much more potent method of avoiding further painful therapeutic work in the inpatient setting where the therapist is ofen viewed as a "super-parent" who can be angered, humiliated, or distanced by rejecting or disrupting the small universe that the therapist directs and controls, namely the inpatient treatment unit. In other words, the entire hospital situation may come to represent the therapist and thereby provide a broad stage for "acting-in" an extended trans-ference image.

It is obvious that dramatic events of this kind signal a disruption of the therapeutic alliance. They are drastic actions which are de-signed to force the therapist to assume some role with the patient aside from that of neutral therapeutic guide. The patient may be courting rejection to avoid a frightening growing closeness, eliciting greater concern and protectiveness to evade the unwanted psycho-logical equality offered in the alliance, or tempting the therapist to a position of anger which can be eroticized in sadomasochistic fash-ion. Although forces of this kind are almost always in operation when a relatively smooth therapeutic course is interrupted by a dramatic event, there is rarely a good opportunity to interpret the meaning of the action in the period of time immediately following its occurrence. Since the alliance has been disrupted, the treatment situation itself is not ripe for genuine acceptance of interpretations.

In addition, the chaos created in staff and family usually leads to a variety of theories regarding the youngster's motivation, most of which reflect the anger which the patient has stirred. For example, if the prevalent theory among the nursing staff is that the youngster went AWOL in order to "show off" and appear a hero to his fellow patients, the therapist's notion that the patient went AWOL because his growing affection for the therapist raised fears of homosexual attachment is likely to be viewed as psychiatric nonsense. In fact, the therapist may be accused of being hoodwinked by his young patient. Nursing staff may feel the therapist is trying to protect the patient from the just consequences of his behavior. It is particularly difficult to make the appropriate interpretation convincingly when the youngster's behavior during and after the AWOL fits the staff's description rather precisely. The issue is even more clouded if the patient himself agrees that he ran away to prove that he could get away with it or "just for the hell of it." In inpatient treatment it is particularly important to work backward from observable behavior and to raise questions which may permit both staff and patient to expand their understanding of the multiple causations of a particular act. In the example described above, the therapist may agree that the youngster was "showing off" but may raise thoughtful questions about why he might have particular needs at the present time to demonstrate his bravery, contempt for authority, and resourcefulness. In both therapy sessions and staff meetings it may gradually become clear to everyone that the youngster's behavior was a counterphobic defensive action.

In the effort to decipher the meaning of acting-out, it is also very valuable to observe the patient's expectations of the therapist's response. Has he anticipated that the therapist would punish him, criticize him, withdraw affection from him or, conversely, does he expect that the therapist will now realize that the patient's complaints about the hospital were really serious and take better care of him? Often the patient does not verbalize expectations but shows in his behavior an anticipation of altered responses from the therapist. Commenting on these expectations may lead to a fruitful discussion of those transference feelings which disrupted the therapeutic alliance.

Of course, some youngsters act out in a way so dangerous to themselves, staff or other patients, or to the design of the treatment program, that continued psychotherapy becomes dangerous or impractical. However, before deciding that this is objectively the case, one must consider carefully the countertransference feelings which exist in both the therapist and the nursing staff. As a rule of thumb, unless one can honestly say that the decision that the youngster is untreatable is a reluctant and sad one, there is a good possibility that the staff may be acting out its anger, disappointment, or sadistic wishes toward the patient.

Alliance with Parents

There is a final area which must be considered in discussing the therapeutic alliance in the inpatient treatment of adolescents. It was mentioned earlier that the therapist treating an adolescent must maintain an alliance with the patient's parents. This is even more true in the case of inpatient treatment. However, the alliance is extremely difficult to gain and maintain when a youngster is hospitalized. There is a massive family regression when adolescents are placed in inpatient therapy. In this situation the parents frequently identify with their adolescent youngster and demonstrate toward the hospital staff the same attitudes and complaints that their youngster had previously demonstrated toward them. The parents project onto the treatment center staff all of the parental deficiencies which have occasioned such guilt in them. Obviously this psychological state of affairs makes it quite difficult to establish an objective working alliance. The exact expression of the parental attitude varies greatly across individual families. Some parents show an exaggerated helplessness and passive compliance while other parents react with a querulous, fault-finding animosity which the staff tends to find exasperating.

Finding ways to help the parents to regain their best level of adult functioning and, in fact, to improve on it is a crucial undertaking.

The parents enjoy a new opportunity to reestablish themselves as important people in the adolescent's emotional life in the course of a youngster's hospitalization. Ideally, parents will accept the responsibility for the inpatient placement and its continuation. Rather than saying, "We'd love to have you home as soon as Dr. Jones says you're ready," the family can state clear expectations regarding the youngster's behavior and his readiness to resume appropriate functioning in a family setting. Obviously, this is helpful not only to the process of reestablishing sensible generational boundries but in psychotherapy. Rather than having to function as a benevolent jailer who spends massive amounts of energy and time convincing both parents and youngster that the child should not return home until treatment goals are reached, the therapist can function in the role of an objective expert whose goal is to assist the family toward living successfully with one another as soon as possible. Naturally, this does a great deal to cut down on the use of confinement as an extraneous resistance issue in inpatient adolescent treatment.

The Inpatient Staff

The nursing care staff and educational staff in an adolescent inpatient treatment unit frequently have a somewhat thankless job. On balance they frustrate the adolescent patient much more frequently than they gratify him. Since they are entrusted with the education of young people who have frequently developed extremely negative attitudes toward school, these staff members cannot afford even the limited degree of permissiveness which the therapist can permit in his inpatient psychotherapy sessions. Frequently they are the "bad guys" who do not "understand"—namely that the patient is behaving badly because he is angry, anxious, or in desperate need of a rebellious stance. They cannot afford to "understand" these issues since they must insist on a minimal level of behavioral expectation. In spite of the surging torrent of emotions and impulses which are stirred in the patients by the treatment process, nursing and teaching staff must reinforce ego control. They are the keepers of reality's demands.

Because of these circumstances in hospital treatment, the opportunities for "splitting" abound. The patient may appear to have a warm and cooperative therapeutic relationship with the primary therapist while continuing to act out the negative side of his ambivalence with other staff members in an unexamined and guilt-free way. Needless to say, a pseudo-alliance of this kind does not actually benefit the patient since important areas of psychopathology are excluded from the treatment process and expressed uncritically in everyday life on the unit.

The patient's tendency to split in this way may easily be reinforced by unexpressed and unexamined splits between the various staff members. Therapists frequently view nursing staff as controlling and insensitive to dynamic treatment issues. Nursing staff may view therapists as overly permissive and naive regarding the patient's genuine motives. The educational staff is frequently the object of resentment. Nursing staff is frequently extremely jealous of school holidays which regularly rekindle the chronic suspicion that teachers have a much easier life than they do. Therapists often view teachers as inflexible and overly concerned with the youngster's cognitive development and conventional educational expectations at the expense of emotional growth. Perhaps all staff members carry consciously or unconsciously some of the fear and resentment of teachers which most of us develop during our personal educational experiences. These negative memories make it easy to identify with the adolescent patient's hostility toward the teaching staff.

It is the responsibility of the therapist to understand and appreciate the contributions made by all disciplines and to recognize the interdependence of the entire treatment team. Opportunities for discussion of tensions and conflict between staff members must be provided so that the patients are not used to act out staff problems.

In direct work with the patient, it is crucial to insist on generalizing the therapeutic alliance. For example, the question of confidentiality in inpatient psychotherapy frequently provides a clue to the real strength of the alliance. Many patients try to create splits between the therapist and the remainder of the staff by offering to share information if the therapist will promise to keep it secret from nursing or teaching staff. As a rule, much more is lost than gained by making such promises. Of course, the therapist frequently makes choices regarding the kind of psychotherapy material which can be fruitfully shared with the extended staff. Often it is disruptive rather than helpful to discuss a patient's fantasies, dreams, and transference interactions in great detail with the staff. This is basically intrapsychic information which has its primary value in the one-to-one treatment situation. On the other hand, overt actions, interactions with other patients, family issues, and aspirations in the real world are important data for the entire staff to consider. Not only should the therapist insist on the freedom to use his own judgment in sharing material from individual psychotherapy, but he should strongly encourage the patient to share sensitive information with other staff members so that the alliance is generalized and its gains are moved closer to ordinary daily living. That is, if the patient can discuss distorted attitudes and conflicts with the staff members whom he lives with 24 hours each day, he is one step closer to the capacity for self-observation and self-direction in ordinary family life and social interactions outside the home.

The therapist needs to also be alert to the relationships that the inpatient adolescent has with fellow patients. A fragmentation of emotional experience, similar to that seen in relationships with staff, may occur in relationships with fellow patients. Intensive positive or negative interaction with other youngsters in the treatment program may represent the true focus of the patient's emotional investment, leaving the therapeutic alliance empty and bland though apparently constructive.

The patient may also utilize fellow patients to act out conflicts by proxy, collude with them in the avoidance of significant emotional issues, or use them to bolster up defenses in other ways. This is not to say that the therapist attempts to thwart these intense interpatient interactions. This would be an impossible task and probably not desirable in any event. However, it is important to be aware of what is happening among the adolescents on the unit so that these issues can be effectively addressed in the treatment. The therapist must usually depend on the observations of nursing and educational staff members for this data since the patient is unlikely to report them in therapy for obvious reasons.

SUMMARY

The therapeutic alliance is the key to effective psychotherapy. Original discussions of the alliance were strongly influenced by the model of psychoanalysis. This basic model is frequently adequate for outpatient dynamic psychotherapy and should always serve as an ideal endpoint for any therapeutic relationship. However, it does seem possible in some instances to permit and encourage psychological growth through relationships which show considerable variation from an objective alliance based on a mutual commitment to understanding the patient's psychological functioning. Obviously, this is an area that we have only begun to explore.

The therapeutic alliance in inpatient treatment is more complex, richer, and more likely to erupt in dramatic acting-out (or acting-in) behavior than the alliance observed in outpatient treatment. These problems are offset by the wealth of information available to the therapist in the inpatient setting if the therapist is able to maintain a reasonably smooth and collaborative working relationship with the remainder of the staff.

REFERENCES

ADATTO, C. P. On the metamorphosis from adolescence into adulthood. *J. Am. Psychoanal. Assoc.*, 14:485-509, 1966.

AICHHORN, A. *Wayward Youth*. New York: Meridian Books, 1935.

FRIEDMAN, L. *The Therapeutic Alliance. Int. J. Psycho-Anal.*, 50:139-153, 1969.

GIOVACCHINI, P. The difficult adolescent patient: Countertransference problems. *Adolescent Psychiat.*, 3:271-288, 1974.

JOHNSON, A. M. Sanctions for superego lacunae of adolescents. In K. R. Eissler (Ed.), *Searchlight on Delinquency*. New York: International Universities Press, Inc., 1965.

KEITH, C. R. The therapeutic alliance in child psychotherapy. *J. Am. Acad. Child Psychiatry*, 7:31-43, 1968.

KERNBERG, O. *Borderline Conditions and Pathological Narcissism*. New York: Aronson, 1975.

KOHUT, H. *The Analysis of the Self*. New York: International Universities Press, Inc., 1971.

LEWIS, J. M., GOSSETT, J. T., KING, J. W., & CARSON, D. *Development of a Pro-Treatment Group Process Among Hospitalized Adolescents*. Timberlawn Foundation Report No. 40, 1970.

MEEKS, J. E. Behavior disorders. In Joseph Noshpitz (Ed.), *The American Handbook of Child Psychiatry*. New York: Basic Books, in press.

MEEKS, J. E. *The Fragile Alliance: An Orientation to the Outpatient Psychotherapy of the Adolescent*. Baltimore: The Williams and Wilkins Co., 1971. (Reprinted by the Robert E. Krieger Publishing Co., Huntington, New York, 1973.)

MEEKS, J. E. Homesickness and the Homesickness Crisis in Residential Therapy. *J. Amer. Acad. Child Psychiatry*, 7:296-315, 1968.

9

Individual Psychotherapy with Adolescents

EDWIN S. KESSLER, M.D.

Not too long ago psychotherapy meant *individual* therapy. The earliest efforts with adolescents were slight modifications of the psychoanalytic method (Klein, 1950). Results were not impressive; the obstacles to therapy were obvious, but the study of these obstacles led to increased knowledge about adolescent development. Some of the problems noted were the reluctance of adolescents to permit dependency, outright suspicious rejection of adults, the increase of narcissism at the expense of object relations, and the tendency to discharge tension through impulsive acting-out rather than through verbalization and reflective endeavor (Fraiberg, 1955, Geleerd, 1957). Furthermore, parental support for continuing therapy was required in the face of the adolescent's ability to stir up disturbing and passionate reactions in all the adults involved.

In time, alternatives to individual therapy for all patients were sought for economic reasons, because of failure of existing methods and out of broadened attempts to understand and modify human behavior. With adolescents, more than with any other age group, the search for different therapeutic approaches was motivated by the sense of complete frustration of attempts to establish or maintain a therapeutic alliance with so many of them. As early as 1925, Aichhorn recognized that major modifications of techniques were required to engage the adolescent in therapy.

In the past 20 to 25 years, knowledge about adolescents has increased tremendously and a wide variety of psychotherapeutic techniques is now available. The challenge for the psychiatrist today is to determine the most suitable approach or combination of therapies. It is certainly true that the availability and sophistication of newer methods, such as group therapy, family therapy, pharmacotherapy, combined with special schools, group homes, treatment centers and adolescent hospital units, have made treatment possible for a broad range of adolescent patients. Basic to all these strides in treatment of adolescents has been the less dramatic but remarkable expansion of our knowledge of adolescent development in each of its phases. With this knowledge, the use of the various modalities singly or in combination offers more possibilities for effective work.

A clinician may face a dilemma of choice when he is particularly skilled and partial to one mode of treatment while seeing possible indications for another. A clinician who works only with individuals may hesitate to refer a patient for family or group therapy when it is not clear that individual therapy has a poor prognosis. A consultant who is responsible for the treatment plan needs to recognize the validity of different modalities, to be able to assess the relative indications, and to guide the patient and his family toward a proper choice.

How does one make this assessment? Neither the diagnostic label nor the severity of the symptoms is a clear indicator. Especially with adolescents, two issues predominate. One issue has to do with the phase of development, especially the level of object relations attained and the current stance of the ego in its struggle to relinquish the intensity of old object ties; at different stages, individual, group or family therapy may have particular advantages or disadvantages. The other issue concerns the degree and kind of family pathology. Resolution of adolescent problems without appropriate family involvement may fail in the presence of strong needs to maintain the undifferentiated family ego, the inability of the mother to permit individuation, the choice of the adolescent to act out unconscious parental drives, projective identification, scapegoating, etc. Positive indications for family and group therapy will be discussed elsewhere.

At this point it should prove useful to focus on the problems and the advantages of individual therapy in relation to phases of adolescent development.

ADOLESCENT DEVELOPMENT AND THE CHOICE OF
TREATMENT MODALITY

Successful negotiation through each stage of development is dependent upon satisfactory progress through the previous stages. For the individual to progress normally through early adolescence, one needs to assume successful consolidation of psychological growth during the latency period. Peter Blos (1962) has pointed out that this in turn requires at least partial resolution of the earlier age-appropriate oedipal conflicts.

The achievements of latency prepare the youngster to handle the changes of puberty. Increased control over sexual and aggressive impulses is due to the growth and expansion of ego and superego. This has taken place with maturation of ego functions leading to increased mastery over the environment, and through wider identifications. Instinctual energy can now be more effectively channeled into cognitive and social growth.

Not many individuals reach preadolescence in an optimal state of development. Nevertheless, the healthier the individual, the more effectively he will handle the sudden influx of instinctual drives at puberty. Relative failure of ego and superego expansion in latency increases the likelihood of a stormy and pathological adolescence.

In most adolescents, the increase of instinctual tension is sufficiently great to interfere with the balance of control by ego and superego and lead to disruption of the psychic organization. Normal adolescents will progress to maturity and reorganization of psychic structure with anywhere from minimal to somewhat dramatic evidence of turmoil.

Daniel and Judith Offer (1976), studied a group of carefully selected normal male adolescents from the beginning of high school through the college years. By observing this non-psychiatric population they found that the psychoanalytic picture of the typical adolescent as moody, impulsive and disturbed in his object relations is characteristic only of the group they termed "tumultuous." Based on observable external behavior, normal adolescents seemed equally divided between "tumultuous," "surgent," and "continuous" growth patterns.

Especially when previous development has been irregular, the adolescent responds to the increased libidinal tension by an urgent effort to withdraw his emotional investment from his early love objects, his parents. The increased involvement with self that results can lead to painful tensions, especially if he does not have other relationships available on which to redirect some of his drives. At this time there can be a deep sense of loneliness and emptiness; not only has the adolescent withdrawn from his actual parents, but he has also rejected their internal representations, the superego. With the absence of these familiar sources for self-esteem, he must turn elsewhere. How well or how soon, or towards whom he will turn is determined by a multitude of factors. The outcome is crucial, and failure or maladaptive efforts can be disastrous.

A goal of adolescent development is to establish mature heterosexual relationships freed from constricting oedipal and pre-oedipal elements. There are times when individual psychotherapy is essential to free the youngster for such progressive development.

Unfortunately, there is no schema of normal and pathological development that would enable the clinician to organize significant variables and then to determine exactly when individual therapy would be regressive and when it would be supportive—or that at a particular point, recommending group therapy would offer wider identifications, freedom from constricting superego, and avoidance of the regressive pull of dependency on an important adult—or that a particular youngster is confronting continuous powerful demands from the family system at a time when no effort on the part of a therapist can help him achieve an independent identity.

The complexities are too involved for a set of handy facts and rules. The adolescent psychiatrist still needs to rely heavily on the inner amalgam of knowledge and intuition. I would like to illustrate, with examples, some of the principles and problems involved in early, midle, and late adolescence. These examples will include difficulties and failures of individual psychotherapy, as well as successful intervention. A secondary intent is to demonstrate, through these examples, flexibility in case management (GAP, 1973). Shifts of treatment plan, work with parents, use of other facilities, out-of-home placement and medication will be mentioned as modes of flexibility.

Early Adolescence

The increase of sexual and aggressive drives in early adolescence is directed at the same objects that were important in latency, but now the manageable equilibrium is disrupted and the drives threaten to break through. The increased strivings towards the early love objects are in conflict with fear, shame, and positive strivings toward independence. The stronger the regressive yearnings, the more forceful may be the rebellion and the rejection of all adults. A kindly, understanding, maternally-perceived therapist may be considered a great danger. The threat of regression implicit in individual therapy may increase the fear of going crazy and bring about an active, hostile refusal of any psychological exploration. Less threatened youngsters at this stage may not be overtly hostile, but still quite suspicious, insisting that they have no need for therapy. The only "help" they seek involves gratification from the environment. Still others may simply be indifferent to an evaluation; they have a sense of adequate security at home and are developing stronger, more satisfactory relationships with peers. In the face of temporary difficulties, they might well accept therapy, provided such help is not culturally unacceptable. They might be brought for therapy because of parental problems with adolescent development, and agree to use the time as a way of negotiating with parents.

Case Report

The case of Jill is an example of the difficulties in establishing an alliance at this age, and of the need to be flexible in use of resources in the evolution of a treatment program. At the time of evaluation she was almost 12 and starting seventh grade in junior high school. At home she was provocative, hostile and demanding toward both parents, but very dependent on her mother, with whom there was a strong, ambivalent bond. Father was mostly remote, but when arguments heated up, he would become enraged at Jill's behavior and beat her. She was, nevertheless, active at school, did well in her studies and seemed to have a number of girlfriends.

The parents fought with each other, and after one of many blow-ups involving Jill, she developed somatic symptoms and, soon afterward, a full-blown stubborn school phobia. Her ability to control the family was phenomenal. When told she had to stay home all day if she did not go to school, she stopped seeing her friends, apparently without regret. When a visiting teacher came to the house and coaxed Jill from her room to the top of the stairs, Jill threw a glass of water at her. She was brought for evaluation by her parents, but she made it clear she was not crazy and would not talk about problems. She sat sullenly by the door and during the third session threatened to scream continuously if asked any more questions. At home she denied her dependency with loud protestations of hostility and contempt. Onset of menarche occurred during this evaluation, but with no apparent upset to Jill or her mother.

The impasse was broken by hospitalization on a pediatric ward. The therapist visited her there explaining she did not have to return to school at this point, but she had to accept certain conditions in order to return home: schooling and therapy. The therapist acknowledged that she might very well prefer another therapist; she surprised him by saying he probably knew more about the whole situation and she would come to his office.

For a variety of reasons, including transference and countertransference situations, therapy with a woman therapist was arranged. She established a tolerable alliance with Jill, but the family pathology was so severe that it was barely possible for any member to feel safe from violence. After two months of work with Jill and her parents, it became apparent that relief from the struggle was essential. The parents accepted the recommendation of a residential treatment center for Jill and therapy for themselves.

A second example will illustrate relatively rapid progress in individual therapy because this post-pubertal youngster had not yet entered psychological adolescence.

Case Report

Stanley, almost 14, was brought by his disapproving, success-driven parents because of his poor grades in school, passive-aggressive behavior at home, and annoying teasing of his older and younger sisters. Father was a prosperous dentist, proud of his academic honors and monetary success. His distaste and contempt for Stanley were obvious. Mother appeared sugary sweet, but was clearly hostile and critical of her husband, son, father and brother. All arguments among the children were attributed to Stanley's provocations, never to his older sister. Stanley did not want therapy and denied all problems. He smiled sweetly, sat with hands folded and said his parents were justified in depriving him of orchestra, band, etc., until his grades improved.

What was different here was that the early adolescent defiance and rejection of the therapist collapsed easily. His passivity and inner need for adult approval, his good intelligence and rapidly developing psychological-mindedness won him over to therapy. It was the parents who ended therapy abruptly despite the collaborative work they were doing with a colleague and despite Stanley's wish to continue. They acknowledged Stanley had improved greatly but, since he was nine months older, they decided he had outgrown his problems. They complained that his therapist just chatted with him, and in some ways therapy had caused more trouble because he was now analyzing everyone's motives. After a four-way conference, they agreed to continue therapy for three months longer since the original time estimate had been for at least one year. Stanley and his therapist worked through the separation as much as possible and reviewed the gains. They agreed there was more to do but that he was now in a better position to handle the family view of him without total resort to self-defeating mechanisms. The therapist had great difficulty in steering a course between confronting Stanley with his continuing problem of passivity, allowing him to see the reality of his scapegoating parents, and avoiding destructive criticism of them.

Here, early adolescence was chiefly in chronology. In terms of dependency, or expression of drive, Stanley was more like a child in latency. With therapy, he made considerable gains in ego competence, developed some assertiveness, and attained better reality-testing, Still, ego and superego structures were not sufficiently enlarged. Group therapy alone would not have offered the adult support needed to begin to relinquish dependent ties; conjoint therapy would probably have been rejected even more vigorously than the program provided, although clearly the failure to enlist family support became the major problem. It is theoretically possible that a later breakthrough of rebellion or manifest neurosis may have mobilized the family to seek further treatment with someone else. There has not been a follow-up. The issue here is not that this early adolescent boy who initially refused therapy should have been treated by group or family therapy. The fact is that individual therapy was appropriate and that substantial gains were made. The therapy was prematurely interrupted, possibly due to some misjudgment in the setting up of the original treatment plan, or in countertransference problems the therapist had with the parents.

The more nearly a youngster has progressed in his development to preadolescence, the more useful phase-appropriate, valued peer relationships can be in therapeutic intervention. Where individual therapy may be actively rejected, group therapy can dilute the dangers of the transference and offer peer support, along with alternative solutions to current conflicts. When ego structure is fairly intact but under the pressure of unusually severe oedipal conflicts, individual therapy may be necessary to bring development along, into, and through latency. On the other hand, it is possible that the youngster still struggling with pre-oedipal problems of lack of individuation and enmeshed in continuing pathological family relationships will have the greatest need for family therapy.

Mid-Adolescence

Mid-adolescence may present a very different picture. At this phase of development the adolescent may have vigorously rejected his need for parental support. In addition, he has withdrawn cathexis from the internal representation of his oedipal and preoedipal figures as well. He has made some attempt to establish peer relationships, but a sense of discontinuity from his former self causes him to feel isolated and depressed. As described earlier, the absence of former sources for self-esteem requires that some important relationship be established.

Case Report

This development phase of mid-adolescence can be illustrated by the case of Valerie, who was 14½ years old when referred by her family doctor. She was beginning the tenth grade in a suburban high school. Her defiant, hostile attitude toward her parents, especially her mother, had the household in a turmoil. From a very wealthy, but conventional middle-class family, Valerie completely rejected the style, appearance and values of her family and joined up with the activist, hippie subculture. Arguments were incessant about clothing, cutting school, lack of studying, hitchhiking, unkempt hair, bad companions and, finally, drugs. The parents were frightened that the child was now completely out of control and would influence her two younger brothers. Her older sister, a senior in high school, was attractive, popular, fairly independent, but adaptable.

From having encountered similar situations, the therapist anticipated massive resistance to individual therapy, and a probable need for family therapy, or even out-of-home placement. Nevertheless, the first interview was with Valerie, partly because she agreed to the interview, and partly because of the parents' underlying naive expectation that Valerie would come as a patient, be treated, and behave reasonably. She was an angry, but rather vulnerable-looking girl with long, light brown hair and a soft, rounded face. She was determinedly anti-establishment, pro dropouts, freaks and any kind of political activism. She represented a surprising mixture of angry complaints, idealistic cliches, and highly perceptive observation about herself and her parents.

The parents were seen during the initial evaluation and thereafter about twice a month. At first the therapist was concerned that this would identify him as supporting the parents' expectations as a goal of therapy. It seemed not to have occurred to Valerie. Surprisingly, she almost immediately took on two responsibilities: to come regularly and to report about all of her activities, including those she knew were considered dangerous—indiscriminate hitchhiking, smoking pot during the week, and any use of hard drugs. For a while, she continued to smoke marijuana daily, sleep in class or cut school altogether, provoke her parents, and encourage her friends to do so. She would then become indignant and retaliatory when the parents were punitive. The parents claimed she had completely changed, cared for no one but herself, was a liar, and was destroying their home. Mother said, "I have ulcers, can stand it no longer; one of us has to go." Father was more resilient, but felt he had to support mother.

Valerie was presented to the parents as a deeply dependent girl who felt so close to her mother that she could only escape from her dependency by total denial. The therapist wanted them to see her as basically warm-hearted and sentimental, rather than cold and selfish; as freshly attractive instead of shamefully ugly; and as struggling toward a healthy, self-approving individuality. Mother found the meetings upsetting, sometimes made lame excuses not to come, sometimes frankly acknowledged through father she "couldn't take it." After a few months, Valerie said that things at home, which had improved for a while, were worse again. She urged the therapist to insist on more frequent parental visits. She knew that he was not mediating any arguments or struggles over rules, but perceived, probably accurately, that her parents were more openly derogatory and confronting when they missed appointments.

Valerie and her parents were seen for over two years through a variety of family, school and peer group crises. For a while parents came weekly, but father was often alone. At a particular point in her therapy, where Valerie was struggling with some bisexual problems, but moving clearly toward heterosexuality, she decided she had to proceed further without the help of therapy. The therapist concurred, but continued to see the parents for a period after her termination, which, incidentally, he really considered to be a developmental interruption.

Basically, things had gone very well. Why? Valerie was depressed and frightened at the road she had taken. Walled off from her parents by her own removal from them, she found no real kinship with the rebellious groups she drifted into and out of. For a while she worked with the May Day group and then joined a women's commune in which numerous members had already left home and dropped out. She was defensive to her friends and even to her therapist about her inability to be truly liberated and to have a loving sexual relationship with her girlfriend; then she fell in love with a boy who had joined the Gay Liberation Party. She decided to leave school after the tenth grade but, with some support, agreed to attend a permissive boarding school not too distant from home.

Several near disasters were avoided by supporting the parents' ability to permit compromise. In an almost counterphobic way, they sometimes threatened to reject Valerie from the household in order to avoid the feeling of helplessness engendered by her rebelliousness. Gradually she established and asserted her own values, truly incorporating aspects from school, peer group, therapist and even parents. Three years later it was learned through a chance meeting with her parents that Valerie was studying the anthropology of dance at a small college in California and that all three had arrived at a very happy relationship with each other. The distance helped, but visits home were really enjoyable.

The focus was on Valerie as a patient and the concern was for the evolution of a strong, independent ego with its creative potential available. The other siblings were not seen, but the therapist did intervene in the family system to reduce the stress on Valerie and her parents. In the course of this, the father assumed an increasingly dominant role and there was some positive change in the family. It went well, not just because the treatment was supported with work with the family, which child psychiatry has always done, but because Valerie had a very special need. She had to reject her mother totally because the symbiotic pull was too threatening. Full of bravado, she plunged uncritically and superficially into relationships with the most rebellious groups and denied any anxiety about her risky activities. At this point she was in combat with her parents, isolated from her superego, feeling a sense of discontinuity from her past self, with no ability to sustain affective attachment to peers or embrace the group superego for self-esteem regulation.

Through her psychiatrist she was not completely cut off from her parents or the internal representation of them and she could use him almost as a transitional object between her old self and the unfamiliar new self and new object. He provided a permissible, unacknowledged but void-filling affective relationship. It wasn't until the second-to-last session at age 17 that she said clearly, "It's time I stopped coming to tell you everything like you were a diary. I've been very dependent on you." At this midpoint in adolescence, individual psychotherapy for Valerie, as for many adolescents, serves a development need.

Late Adolescence

Frequently, the indications for and techniques of psychotherapy with late adolescents are much like those with young adults. There are, however, some advantages for the therapist in working with late adolescents. There is more "plasticity"—that ability of the psyche to alter structure that has not yet taken definitive form. It is also true that consolidation of psychic structure leading to a clear sense of identity with healthy ego-ideal formation is the task of this period.

Psychopathology, whether long-standing or arising in adolescence, can interfere with this development process. The therapist does function in his traditional role as representative of reality vs. primary process thinking and unconscious regressive drive motivation. However, his availability as a model for identification and for ego-ideal consolidation takes on a relatively greater dimension because of the phase-specific needs of the late adolescent. It is in this period that severe upheavals occur in the pathologically structured ego; the subsequent reorganization can be crucial. Individual psychotherapy at this time offers more possibility of success than chance outcome alone.

Case Report

Jeff was a 19-year-old who dropped out of a midwestern college after two weeks in order to attempt a reconciliation with his girlfriend at another university. His high school grades were slightly above average but he had been recognized as a bright student with a flair for literature and poetry. He was also a good athlete and fairly popular in a small private school run by unconventional educators for unconventional students. After dropping out of college, he returned to his home city and managed to support himself, by tutoring and odd jobs, in an apartment shared with a new girlfriend. The tension of hostile dependency on his girlfriend and lack of direction in work led him to seek weekly psychotherapy.

After six months he abruptly ended therapy and took a job on a freighter to the Orient. He lived in Thailand for a year, studying the language and partially supporting himself by tutoring the son of a wealthy merchant family with which he lived. Oedipal conflicts began to be played out in relation to the family, causing increasing anxiety. He tried to establish control over his bodily sensations through a series of rigorous exercises and meditation. He also became engaged to a Thai girl. She was an airline hostess whose repeated departures from him became intolerable. He thought that her father and brother were plotting to murder him. His psychotic thinking became evident to the host family and his father was called to bring him home. When he was next seen in therapy he was coherent, but suffering from panic states, episodic paranoid delusions and occasional auditory hallucinations which he recognized as such. Regular psychotherapy three times a week was started as soon as possible. Only minor tranquilizers were used, on occasion, for anxiety.

A combination of circumstances led to truly remarkable and rapid reintegration. He was now living at home accepting a degree of dependency; the parents had considerable confidence in the psychiatrist because of work with them some years earlier; and Jeff had had previous psychotherapy with him. His earlier abrupt termination had been due to external circumstances rather than primary flight from treatment, with which he was not deeply involved.

This time he took on psychotherapy as a life preserver and a challenge. He found employment as a carpenter's apprentice and delighted in the opportunity to work with his hands in precise, orderly ways. He cautiously returned to college, taking two courses; then he decided he would do better with full enrollment. The therapy, after nine months, shifted from psychotherapy to psychoanalysis. His progress was remarkable; it seemed as though he was reorganizing his life from within and the analysis removed obstacles. After another year he was supporting his analysis with part-time work and insurance. He graduated from the university with high honors and was accepted into a prestigious doctoral program. Treatment was terminated at this point by mutual consent. By this time he was financially self-sufficient except for tuition and had married a young woman student who was also working and finishing her B.S. degree.

In his second year of graduate school. he returned to analysis, but it was clear that the intense conflicts that had erupted at adolescence, causing an acute psychotic disorganization of the ego, were no longer a major threat. Previous to his breakdown his energies had been directed toward repression, displacement and flight. The reorganization of psychic structure that occurred following his psychosis had, with the help of psychotherapy, permitted a stability of perception and function that assisted his further development. A major factor in his healthier reintegration and mobilization of his energies for analytic work was his intense need for a consistently approving, non-competitive father figure.

In analytic terms, the resolution of the negative oedipal conflict (the longing for love and approval from the parent of the same sex) is a major task of late adolescence (Blos, 1974). It is accomplished by recognition of and subsequent relinquishing of these wishes. This occurs through gradual assimilation into the self of those aspects of the parent and his surrogates that can be incorporated into a realistic ego-ideal.

SPECIAL CONSIDERATIONS IN TECHNIQUE

Assisting the adolescent to master his developmental tasks and make successful progress through the successive stages of adolescence is the primary goal of psychotherapy. By late adolescence it is hoped that the individual has been able to relinquish his early ties to nurturing adults and establish mature heterosexual relationships. Further progress toward ego mastery with beginning establishment of a work identity has occurred, along with modification of the primitive superego. Finally, in late adolescence the establishment of a realistic ego-ideal provides a direction for adult strivings.

In some instances there is need for preliminary work to bring development up to psychological adolescence. With this emphasis in overall strategy, this chapter has demonstrated that the individual's developmental needs, as well as the degree and kind of family pathology, may determine the choice of individual psychotherapy as the predominant mode.

There are also special considerations in what, by analogy, might be considered the tactics of psychotherapy. The special problems of establishing and maintaining a therapeutic alliance are discussed in Chapter 8; these problems are considerably greater with adolescents than with adult patients.

Countertransference Issues

Countertransference issues with adolescents are often more prominent and more easily rationalized than with adults. The therapist must be relatively free from his own adolescent conflicts and have sufficient awareness of them to maintain his objectivity. Especially for younger therapists, it is quite easy to become identified with the adolescent, rebellious with him, and involved in his goals and strivings. This can interfere with his achieving a compatible adjustment to his own family and society.

It is quite possible to recognize the adolescent's wish to free himself from engulfing overrestrictive parents without supporting him uncritically and without endangering the alliance.

Case Report

A 16-year-old high school student told his psychiatrist that his soccer team was playing a school in New York state the next weekend. His family had given him permission to drive five of his teammates from Washington to Baltimore, where they were to pick up a special bus for New York. However, he was planning to drive directly to New York with the family car. He knew that his doctor would not report this information to his parents but that he was concerned about the danger of his plan. The therapist asked him if he felt quite certain that he could withstand the pressures from his five teammates as they engaged in horseplay, teasing, urging him to pass the car ahead, and such—and still keep his cool. He asserted that it would be no problem. The therapist told him he thought it was a considerable risk and worth thinking about. The psychiatrist was surprised to find out the following week that he had decided to leave the car in Baltimore and go by bus. This was particularly interesting because of his frequent complaints of anxious hovering overcontrol by his mother and either stupid indifference or giving way to mother on the part of his father. By the therapist's quietly presenting his own viewpoint for consideration, the young patient was able to consider the reality aspects and separate them from his need to defy his mother and prove his father helpless.

Personal Style and Role of the Therapist

Personal style is important in forging the alliance; it is also useful in ongoing therapy. By "personal style" I am referring to the comfortable, spontaneous use of one's familiar mode of interacting with peers. It is compounded from an amalgam of ego-coping approaches, successful defenses, and learned experiences. It differs from an assumed role such as "non-judgmental, relatively anonymous analyst" who carefully monitors the nature of his interventions, or "wise, older friend" who educates with direct advice as well as by providing a model for identification. Role assumptions can be temporary and are innumerably varied. Often style and role overlap, but style is close to the core of the personality and role is more distant.

Both style and role are employed in any personal interaction. Therapists need to be aware of their role assumptions so as not to be restricted to a narrow range mandated by one obligatory approach. Adolescents are particularly alert to defensive role-playing in adults. To communicate adequately, one must avoid role assumptions such as adult-child, teacher-student, medical authority-patient, or similar protective stance. The reality is that roles will be thrust upon the therapist by way of transference. He must be able to sustain his own concept of the therapist role.

It is my impression that therapists who are fairly successful with adolescents and who enjoy working with them have a personal style that facilitates comfortable interchange without condescension. There is no one mode to recommend; a supervisor of psychotherapy may share his own approach with a trainee psychotherapist, but he should support the trainee in being free to use his own style. The idea of psychotherapy as collaborative therapeutic work then becomes more convincing.

It is also possible for the therapist to be too enamored of the idea that his natural unfettered style is in itself therapeutic. Mental health workers who are relatively untrained with adolescents tend to misuse this concept. They may be aware of their own pleasant experience in being spontaneous, while overlooking the many situations when it is inappropriate. The therapist must be aware of his usual style so that he is also free to *not* use it.

Therapists of widely different personalities can successfully engage the adolescent patient. Being open and friendly may be a relief to the patient who has been neglected by adults and has little hope for recognition by them. However, some are so suspicious that they will perceive the therapist's easygoing manner as a devious maneuver to gain confidence. Friendliness can also be perceived, at times correctly, as the therapist's need to be liked and to deflect anger. This obviously would interfere with the therapeutic process.

A therapist who is comfortable in revealing some personal information and feelings may be providing a very meaningful experience of trust and closeness. But the therapist must be discriminating in the use of this approach. There are times when the adolescent needs to maintain the therapist as a projected, idealized self and is not ready to see him as a human being.

A non-judgmental, non-directive approach may stem from the therapist's tolerance for independent discovery and from his expectation that growth comes from inner awareness. This may be of great use to an adult with good ego controls and too much repression. For many adolescents it will be perceived as a sanction for acting out of the impulses they are struggling to master. However, it is possible to be non-critical while pointing out the reality consequences, as illustrated earlier with the example of the soccer team trip.

Lightly cynical banter, when part of the therapist's usual style, can be enjoyed by therapist and patient. It can defuse a feeling of tension and allow defenses to be challenged without loss of face. The underlying assumption is "we both know what's going on and can see it with perspective." The therapist must also know when to avoid banter so as not to play into the defense of avoiding affect or of devaluing a serious feeling.

Most therapists tend to be serious, considerate and thoughtful in manner. This style conveys respect and esteem to the adolescent patient and is certainly a valuable therapeutic tool, hardly one to consider with suspicion. But some adolescents can even manage that; they will be hostile to such an approach, seeing it as stuffiness or an emphasis on the obvious. In such instances, the alliance may be more difficult to achieve than with the therapist who uses humor. Sometimes the personality fit is worth considering. Also, the therapist who has a greater range of style can do well with a wider range of adolescent personalities.

Another type is the "kind uncle." Such a tendency may be a good beginning approach. One shows consideration, sympathy, willingness —even readiness—to answer questions and give advice. If one has this tendency, it is important to recognize it and use it with caution. The "kind uncle" can become condescending. By contrast, the therapist who is somewhat admiring of the patient and willing to learn from him conveys a feeling to the adolescent of being valued. It may be the first experience the youngster has had with an adult who listens, approves, and even finds him somewhat fascinating. The same cautions apply here as with the "kind uncle." This gets very close to overidentification with projection of idealized aspects of the self onto the adolescent.

Use of style also fades into areas of countertransference involvements in which interventions are influenced increasingly by the needs of the therapist. Two types of countertransference, can be described: One kind is stirred up by the patient's pathology and is likely to be experienced by most people in dealing with him; it is the understanding of this countertransference that can be illuminating and useful in the conduct of therapy. The other kind is that which psychotherapists bring to their patients, particularly certain patients who tend to elicit these reaction patterns. Therapists who work with adolescents must be especially aware of this kind of countertransference. If these reactions are unconscious and obligatory, they can impede or destroy the therapy. At another level, awareness of and measured use of some of these needs can bring energy, commitment and art into work with adolescents.

SUMMARY

This chapter discussed issues in the treatment of adolescents with individual psychotherapy. Due to the availability of a variety of treatment modalities, an attempt was made to highlight positive indications for individual therapy as the treatment of choice with or without concomitant approaches.

Two issues were emphasized. One issue has to do with the phase of development, especially the level of object relations attained and the current stance of the ego in its struggle to relinquish the intensity of old object ties. The other issue concerns the degree and kind of family pathology. Examples were used to illustrate the occasional harmonizing of developmental need with an individual therapeutic relationship, as well as the increased difficulties encountered with individual therapy at other phases of adolescent development or in certain family settings.

Finally, some special technical considerations uniquely valuable in work with adolescents were discussed. The recognition of adjusting technique to the current developmental needs of the patient is essential. The importance of personal style is greater in work with adolescents because of their use of the therapist in the establishment of identity and in the consolidation of a mature ego-ideal. Since personal style and countertransference are closely related, the therapist must be aware of his own style, and have the freedom to not use it.

REFERENCES

AICHHORN, A. *Wayward Youth*. New York: Viking Press, 1935. (Originally published as Verwahrloste Jugend, Internationaler Psychoanalytischer Verlag, Vienna, 1925.)

BLOS, P. Genealogy of the ego-ideal. *The Psychoanalytic Study of the Child*, Vol. XXIX. New York: International Universities Press, 1974, pp. 43-88.

BLOS, P. *On Adolescence*. New York: The Free Press of Glencoe, 1962.

FRAIBERG, S. Some considerations in the introduction to therapy in puberty. *The*

Psychoanalytic Study of the Child, Vol. X. New York: International Universities Press, 1955, pp. 264-296.

GELEERD, E. Some aspects of psychoanalytic technique in adolescence. *The Psycho-* 1957, p. 26.

GROUP FOR THE ADVANCEMENT OF PSYCHIATRY. *From Diagnosis to Treatment: An Ap-analytic Study of the Child,* Vol. XII. New York: International Universities Press, *proach to Treatment Planning for the Emotionally Disturbed Child,* Vol. VIII, Report No. 87, Sept. 1973.

KLEIN, M. The technique of analysis in puberty. In *The Psychoanalysis of Children.* London: The Hogarth Press. Reprinted 1950, pp. 122-141. (Originally published as *Die Psychoanalyse des Kindes,* Internationaler Psychoanalytischer Verlag, Vienna, 1925.)

OFFER, D. & OFFER, J. Three developmental routes through normal male adolescence. In S. Feinstein & P. Giovacchini (Eds.), *Adolescent Psychiatry,* Vol. IV. New York: Aronson, 1976, pp. 121-141.

10

Group Therapy with Adolescents

PAUL S. WEISBERG, M.D.

The ordinary course of a chapter such as this would be to evolve an historical dimension to the subject of group therapy for adolescents, and then to describe the current trends and problems in the field. I will, instead, focus on those elements of group psychotherapy with adolescents which have particular impact, in my judgment, during a period of history in which cultural, familial and expectational sets are breaking down rapidly. To that end, I will discuss the nature of the process of psychotherapy with the adolescent in a group setting, and then treat certain aspects of group utilization by the adolescent in the larger frame of his or her life.

GOALS OF GROUP THERAPY

Berkovitz and Sugar (1975) briefly but cogently list goals or indications for group psychotherapy for adolescents; to them the first aim of the group process for adolescents is to support, assist and confront the adolescent through peer interaction. Second, they conceptualize the group as a major real-life situation in which the adolescent can study and gradually learn how to change his behaviors. Another of the purposes of group therapy is to stimulate for the adolescent new ways of dealing with interpersonal situations and developing new skills of human relations. They feel that the group stimulates new concepts of self and new models of identification for the adolescent; it helps him feel less isolated; it provides him with

172

a feeling of protection from an overwhelming adult while his vulnerability is high, and it allows the swings of rebellion or submission which eventually stabilize into a healthy ambivalent modeling. In addition, I would suggest that group psychotherapy is useful to the adolescent in reconstructing a reliable, consistent, restorative family-replicative environment in which early deprivations can be modified and subsequent patterns of detached behavior can be minimized. Elsewhere in this volume (Chapter 1), I develop this argument at some length and will not bring it from the ground up in this chapter. The point, however, will be discussed briefly below.

Another addition that I would suggest to the Berkovitz and Sugar list is that the areas of skill formation, confidence in authority relations, heterosexual relations, peer relations of all sorts, job approach, and coalescing of aims for adulthood are all developed in a group setting in ways that are difficult to emulate in individual therapy. This point will also be discussed below.

ADOLESCENT DEFENSES IN GROUPS

The defensive operations of the adolescent have as their aim a combination of self-protection and learning. The particular code by which adolescents communicate among themselves, which is often hidden from the adult community, well expresses this combined motive. Adolescents communicate to each other when they are alone by a connotative verbal style that is open-ended, at times poorly defined, with multiple possible meanings. These meanings usually are in opposed sets, so that if one adolescent says to another, "That's neat," the statement may mean that what is being described is good, what is being described is bad, what is being described is scorned, or scorning. The exact meaning is elusive, as the adolescent's communication ordinarily expresses a combination of meanings which his peers have no trouble in understanding, since the argot is age-specific. To adults, however, such communications are confusing and irritating; they may lead the adult to attempt to make the adolescent specify denotative meaning. This mode of communication style represents the adolescent's set of needing to protect as well as wishing to expand. The adolescent is at the same time integrating his perceptions, avoiding being caught with a confrontative rebellious position, and seeking peer approval and support.

Group psychotherapy functions in analogous ways for adolescents as those connotative messages, in that the adolescent in the group wishes to defend, detach, and if necessary isolate himself from a threatening adult authority system that appears to pressure him or her into positions that may not be tenable, or may lead into a trap. But at the same time, the adolescent is seeking to learn, expand and even to conform to model roles which are available to him from the adult community. Patients have said to me often over the years that the difference between a group and a rap session of adolescents without adults present is that the adolescents in the group are more careful, are more restrained, are more wary. But on consideration, the same elements also exist in the adolescents' communications with each other, although at a lower level. The group then serves to highlight this defensive-offensive function so important to psychic growth.

PSYCHOPATHOLOGY IN ADOLESCENCE

What separates the adolescent with identified psychopathology from the "normal" adolescent? The answers are multiple, but useful to identify. One group of adolescents with psychopathology show early psychoses, usually schizophrenic, in which the attained skills of latency are continually eroded by the ambiguity of the perceptions in the affective area. How the world feels about the adolescent, how the level of acceptance is faring—these are very important questions for the adolescent to determine as guidelines for ongoing behaviors, whether those behaviors are in conformity to or in rebellion from the standards identified. To the schizophrenic adolescent, these responses are unreliable, unclear, and ominous. Withdrawal, resort to delusional thinking, and profound regression are frequent in these cases. We must understand that this affliction is genetic in origin, and that the difference that the psychological underpinnings make is between the latent and the overt form of the disease. Certainly this kind of pathology in adolescence is a discrete, medical, pharmacologically modifiable disorder.

Another set of psychopathological reactions in adolescents refers to immaturity of intellectual function. Retardation is another pathological entity which has profound social effects in the adolescent's life. Secondary responses to the retardation are often neurotic. But retardation, too, is a condition which is at least largely biological in origin, and which imposes limitations on the adolescent which are not wholly surmountable through psychological therapy.

A third form of psychopathology in adolescence appears to have the same unalterability at times as the first two conditions described. This psychopathological set has to do with the "bypass phenomenon" in which behaviors express conflict without being processed by the observant ego in the personality. Delinquent behaviors are often associated with this "bypass phenomenon." The individual appears detached from interpersonal connection in therapeutic situations. Many drug abusers fall in this category.

It is my belief that the "bypass" personality is one which has been exposed to certain formative experiences in the first three years of life. Those experiences appear to involve a denial by the mother of the symbiotic tie with the child, a further denial of the child's attempts at rapprochement during the first half of the second year, a favorable response by the mother to the child's motor attempts and autonomy attempts, and a subtle coding that the safest place is out, that the mother and father cannot deal with the child's dependency needs or their own personality issues, and that the stage of primary autonomy around the age of two has attached to it, therefore, not only the developmental energy appropriate to that stage, but also the energy appropriate to the earlier stages of dependent connection with the mothering figure. Therefore, interpersonalization and a sense of adequacy out of interpersonal acceptance, which is so much a part of a normal developmental process, is changed to a solipsistic view of the world, with few interpersonal connections of depth, and a gratification through behaviors which confirm that primary autonomy. These children, by the time they reach adolescence, have a built-in proclivity to physical expression of emotional states. It is not necessary for them to interpersonalize their response, to care very much about the responses of others to their behaviors, and thus they tend to bypass consideration of the interpersonal consequences of the act to be performed. While these adolescents are not psychotic, and are not intellectually retarded, they are difficult to treat in a psychiatric setting because they have no reward systems, or at best few reward systems, which respond to the kinds of pressures available in the therapy. Parenthetically, these behavior disordered adolescents characteristically do better in a group setting in which they have peers who are also behavior disordered, as well as peers who are not burdened with their particular character formation. The reason, I believe, why progress is noted in such group settings is that even these adolescents have the combined needs referred to above for safety and expansion; their fellow behavior disordered peers give them a sense of security and the other peers give them a stimulus to learn and even perhaps to change their character style.

Adolescents who have successfully traversed the first three years of life with only minor bruises and who escape the afflictions of psychosis and retardation become pathological only with greater external stress, and their pathological states are much less persistent. As well as high stress, adolescence offers high opportunity and high excitement, so that the natural human tendency to heal and to restore is more notable perhaps in adolescence than in any later age span in life. There is frequently a feeling in the therapist that this kid did well while in therapy, and probably would have been okay had he not received therapy, although it was hard to determine that at the time therapy was initiated. Adolescents who are suffering from psychological disturbances referent to separation from the securities of childhood, anxieties referent to recrudescent sexual issues in the home, and those whose anxieties center around fears of failure to achieve sufficient skills to be adequate in an adult world—these adolescents are a joy to treat, in that I know that time and natural growth processes are on my side as a therapist. The use of the peer group and the quality of the therapist's personality can hasten recovery for these adolescents; it is fair, I believe to say that any form of therapy is effective for these patients, and that the advantages of the group of these afflicted adolescents is mainly in the easier authority confrontation, economic effectiveness, and space for them to back off at times from transference blockages.

FUNCTIONS OF GROUP THERAPY

The main functions of group psychotherapy with adolescents are to supply a substitute flexible authority, to supply restitutive security so that narcissistic self-destructiveness can be lessened, to train in social affiliative skills, to increase confidence necessary to engage work skills, and, finally, to free the adolescent from residual guilty dependency. Group methods used to further these aims cover a broad range from modified psychoanalytic technique to insight therapy, supportive therapy, situational support, and task-oriented groups devoted to job-finding, drug withdrawal, political radicalization or spiritual enhancement. This chapter will be limited to a discussion of groups that are devoted to the achievement of insight, although much of the tactical expertise available to the group psychotherapist comes out of sociological research which bears on other types of group interaction. A few years ago, for instance, "encounter" groups were popular. These groups achieved their impact through teaching what were, to the participants, revolutionary attitudes relating to tolerance of self and appreciation of others. More commonly, group psychotherapy techniques are evolutionary in their approach style and achieve their effect through repetition, externalization of the problem through seeing it in another, modeling behaviors, and operant conditioning techniques which stress reward for performance and non-punishment for non-performance.

The group, through its stability, value-solidification, acceptance of defensiveness, and encouragement of growth in each adolescent, develops in patients a willingness to achieve solutions to skill deficient problem areas in themselves. Homogeneity as to adolescent stage is very desirable. Kids in an earlier stage than other group members tend to be easily shamed by them, and anything structural in the therapeutic situation that tends to strengthen guilty dependency, evoke inappropriate shame, or isolate the adolescent from the peer group should be avoided, since the overall aim of the therapeutic interaction is to oppose those trends in the patient's life outside of therapy; working through these shame feelings requires an opportunity for resolution which stage distinction makes more difficult.

Group psychotherapy must act to make the external environmental system more consistent. It must aim at inducing an increased credibility of peer group decision-making, leading to greater peer reliance, and it must teach skills of entry into the peer group for the withdrawing adolescent. At the same time, it must help the individual identify the negative peer group, devoted to behavioral excess, as distinguished from the positive peer group. The negative peer group can be identified best by its essential detachment between its members with the only binding force being the oppositional goal; in a positive peer group the binding force is a interpersonal connection among group members. Group psychotherapy must act to help the adolescent alleviate and resolve feelings of guilty dependency, largely through sharing and opening these feelings to peers whose experiences are similar. The therapy must act to make authority more tolerable to the adolescent, to make it easier for the adolescent to see authority in the bifurcated ally-enemy role through increasing the cumulative strength of opposition to the authority in the group, producing thereby a greater sense of equality and self-confidence in the adolescent and permitting the adolescent to explore feelings toward authority rather than to resist that exploration.

THE GROUP LEADER

The tactics of therapy are largely in the hands of the leader. Who should that leader be? My judgments on this are idiosyncratic, but may be of use: In my view, the leader must be willing to be wrong and to be wronged. The leader should possess a voluntary capacity for open boundaires, setting aside syncretic thinking at will, and reassuming it at will. "Tuning in" to the adolescent requires that capacity. The leader should be of a disposition which does not easily tend toward hierarchical or, as the adolescents would put it, "pompous" declarations of principle. The leader should be tricky and clever and open with his tricks and cleverness. The leader must respect the adolescent's private world and, at the same time, aggressively seek to impinge on that world.

The professional level of the leader is not important, except in cases where therapy may be undercut by parental scorn of the leader's credentials if these are not of the highest level of education and in cases where medical contingencies arise which require medical judgment. The leader must be aware continuously of countertransference phenomena, and, I believe, should be analyzed. The leader must possess a sense of the bizarre, as well as humor about the bizarre, since much of the emotional impact on adolescents comes from their perception of the non-adolescent world as a bizarre place to exist.

The leader need not have achieved a spiritual settling or integration within himself in order to be effective with adolescents; the leader's own search is a continuing positive connection for the adolescents in the group. This is not to say that the leader should expose his personal life with any detail; such is the temptation for young group therapists, but is, in the main, best avoided. However, the leader's quest for a higher degree of personal integration should not be kept from the group; definition of the leader's own quest is usually helpful as long as it does not involve transmission of specific details of life pattern. For instance, the group will know whether the leader is married or not. If the leader does not tell them, they will find out from outside sources. Any disruption in the leader's marital life is none of the group's business. The challenge to grow that accompanies that disruption, however, is appropriately communicated to the group in connecting with concerns and comments from the group members. This question of therapist's disclosure has plagued group psychotherapists for many years; it can be, I believe, resolved by the above formula.

COMPOSITION OF THE GROUP

Who should be in the group? As indicated above, groups do best if they are homogeneous for a stage of adolescence. I believe that schizophrenics do best either in a homogeneous group, or as a sprinkling in a non-schizophrenic group. Few therapists in non-institutional situations have sufficient access to patients to have groups that are homogeneous for schizophrenia. Such groups work very well, under proper guidelines (Horowitz and Weisberg, 1966).

Behaviorally disturbed adolescents fit into a group of schizophrenics well, as long as their population is not predominant. Three or four behaviorally disturbed adolescents in a group of eight or nine is, in my experience, about as many as the group can handle.

Mentally retarded adolescents should not be placed in a group that is not homogeneous for them. Their shame level is increased and their symptomatology often exacerbated when they are placed in a group with normally intelligent adolescents.

Within the above limitations the group should be diagnostically open. Gender balance is highly desirable for middle and late adolescent groups and apt for early adolescent groups with the proviso that the leader must expect and tolerate a two-group element in the group interaction. In early adolescence girls will tend to learn more from and interact more with girls and boys with boys.

OPEN VS. CLOSED GROUPS

Should the group be open or closed? Closed groups work very well for late adolescents if the didactic model is followed. Members of a group will be gathered and informed that the group is to last 15 or 18 months. The group membership is to be stable. The leader defines some of the tasks of the early, middle and late phases of the group. Such a group tends to evoke powerful feelings of commitment and importance of the group in the total life pattern of the adolescent.

Patients who are in early and middle phases of adolescence usually do better in open groups where issues of entree are important and traditions are formed which are transmitted to new members. Such a group gives the adolescent more of a feeling of progressing up the ladder than the closed group; further, the early and middle adolescent is, in general, not yet capable of enduring the continuous deep exploration of his motives and defenses in the way that the late adolescent is. With an open group (which is acceptable too for late adolescents), modeling images emerge, largely based on leader cues, in various of the group members; these then serve to act as a platform for other members, from which they can evolve a more extensive view of their life environment.

FREQUENCY OF MEETINGS

How often should the group meet? I am aware that I diverge from the modal opinion on this issue. My belief is that the group must become as important and integrated a part of the life of the adolescent as is feasible within the constraints of other duties and responsibilities. For that reason I prefer to meet with adolescents three times a week for an hour and a half; twice a week is minimal for the achievement of the goals outlined above. The stigma of group therapy as an ancillary and supportive modality has virtually disappeared from the psychiatric profession; the old codes within the profession, it appears to me, were responsible for the continuance of the once-a-week model in group psychotherapy.

ROLE OF THE FAMILY

What is the role of the family? I use family therapy as a frequent accompaniment to the group with early adolescent patients and an occasional accompaniment to the group with middle adolescent patients. For any adolescent patient, the family is interviewed and the patient is interviewed with the family at least once at the outset of therapy and ad hoc during the therapy. Individual sessions with adolescents are used only to attack a block to group interaction in the patient. The patient must perceive the group as the central therapy modality, and use dyadic contact sparingly and for a purpose. Occasionally I will ask an adolescent to see me individually once or twice; occasionally the adolescent will request these individual sessions himself.

WHEN GROUP MEMBERS "GROW UP"

What does one do as a leader when a group's early adolescents grow to middle adolescents or middle adolescents grow to late adolescents? I transfer them, believing in the usefulness of achieving a new standing in a new group for a patient who is dealing with different problems and has completed, as it were, work in the earlier group without achieving sufficient balance for discharge. I have several adolescent groups, so that it is easy for me to effect transfers. Most adolescent group leaders do not have that kind of flexibility built into their practice, particularly if they are practicing outside of an institution. The best option in the hands of a leader who has only one or two groups of adolescents is to use individual therapy as a pause from group interaction as well as a facilitator of consolidation of skills gained in the group. If a group member has been in therapy for two years or so, the therapist might see that patient individually for a period of six months and then return him either to the same group or to a group of young adults if the patient is in the late adolescent range. This can often enhance the ongoing effect of the previous group experience.

TREATMENT TERMINATION

When is a member ready to go? I have found the most useful answer to be that the patient is ready for discharge when able to utilize the peer group effectively. That means that the peers serve to coalesce adolescent positions as against those of the adult world, and they stabilize otherwise anxiety-laden positions. (To the adolescent, almost everything appears risky because his or her experiential base in adult society is low.) When the adolescent can utilize the peer group as a guide to levels of experimentation and as an organizer for his experiential range, then the adolescent is likely to be ready for termination. The particular adaptiveness of group techniques to the adolescent age range depends largely on the utilization of the peer group as therapeutic reinforcement. When the patient is able to use the peer group outside of therapy as guide, reinforcer and stabilizer, then the therapy becomes less of a necessary adjunct. Other guidelines to the timing of termination refer to tolerance of ambivalence, capacity for tenderness, and integration of the group experience into the defensive structures in a specific and yet individualized way.

A group member will often ask whether I would like to see his or her current heterosexual partner with him or her, more or less as a way of gaining a seal of approval, but also as a method of learning better decision-making skills. In the interaction with the group member and his or her friend, which sometimes seems appropriate to accede to, I listen closely to the group member's productions. Often there is a kind of mimicry of principles or even phrases from the therapy experience. That level of comfort—that integration of the style and viewpoint of the therapy and the leader—is, to me, a signal of readiness to terminate.

How does a group therapy end? The last issues for an adolescent patient in group are somewhat different from those for an adult patient. With adults, issues of equality and assumption of adult power and authority tend to dominate the termination months. For adolescents, who because of their age and experience level are not ready yet to assume full equality to a leader, the issues are more those of finishing with neurotic dependencies and substituting a state of respect and at times affection. I have many patients who keep in touch; the list grows longer each year of ex-patients who have married or graduated from a university or accomplished now those things which they not only did not feel capable of even setting for themselves as goals, but also did not want when they were in therapy. These patients have left therapy successfully without the total resolution of transference often achievable in adult therapy. To remain the alternate adult, the quasi-parental roles should not lie too heavy on the shoulders of a group therapist, since successful growth for the patient will involve some continuation of those roles.

DEVELOPMENTAL ISSUES

The developmental patterns that lead to an imperfect sense of certainty in the young child and a lack of optimism and focus on frustration in the adolescent also lead to a susceptibility to corrective emotional experience. The unmet needs of such adolescents can be supplied in large measure by a group in which pseudo-familial interaction exists, but which opposes narcissistic outcomes. Values are inculcated through modeling and peer acceptance. Skill formation is encouraged in academic or occupational areas through reinforcement both by the peer group and directly by the therapist. Bonding through trust occurs with the willingness of the therapist to be wrong and to be wronged without retribution. The capacity for self-understanding rather than a retreat to an obsessive idealism is enhanced, primarily by the peer group's reinforcement of the group member's trust in the group leader's reliable positive intentions. Pleasurable experience—a moment of tenderness or unexpected acceptance—creates the substrate on which memories are laid down that support the adolescent after the therapy experience is complete. Within the group process such experiences are encouraged and enhanced by the adept group leader.

The group itself has a safe yet flexible boundary. Its major focus is on the processes by which decisions are made rather than on judgments as to the adequacy or inadequacy of the participants' behaviors. In that sense it is a modern institution, training for less boundary-defined, right-wrong patterns of response. At the same time, however, the group is restitutive of traditional securities, in that it gives the adolescent members a chance to develop skills, to introject loving attitudes and to identify with self-confident models, all of which increase hope and enable prudent risk-taking behaviors. The group is a macrocosm of the self and a microcosm of the world around us. It is a social unit with fewer constraints on development than often exist in the adolescent's family. It is an education, a crash course in socialized and interpersonally effective skills. It is research design-sensitive and efficient in the use of the therapist's time and skill. Finally, it is familiar in that it is a family-surrogate institution. The effect of the group can be to establish a baseline of certainty and security, to encourage a non-punitive reexamination of the etiologies, processes, and consequences of behavior, to train in adaptive, non-narcissistic interpersonal relationships, to create a venue for an enhancement of energy for growth that is comparatively free of the fear of frustration, and to diminish the energy tied up in the twin poles of helplessness and omnipotence. Stated another way, the group, through its interpersonal reinforcement and its fulfillment of needs for family-like security, brings the adolescent away from the poles of rage and yearning and toward the desired adult characteristics of adaptiveness, flexibility, and richness of feeling. It aids a solidification of values within the adolescent and restores an emphasis on mastery which childhood experience and training often fail to accomplish in this historical period.

REFERENCES

BERKOVITZ, I. H. & SUGAR, M. Indications and contraindications for adolescent group psychotherapy. In M. Sugar (Ed.), *The Adolescent in Group and Family Therapy.* New York: Brunner/Mazel, pp. 3-26, 1975.

HOROWITZ, M. & WEISBERG, P. Group psychotherapeutic techniques with acute schizophrenics. *International Journal of Group Psychotherapy*, 16 (January):42-50, 1966.

WEISBERG, P. Critical issues in the delivery of group modalities of mental health care to adolescents. In P. Weisberg, (Ed.), *Critical Issues in Adolescent Mental Health.* Washington, D. C.: Metropolitan Washington Society for Adolescent Psychiatry, pp. 87-110, 1978.

11

Adolescents in Family Therapy

ROGER L. SHAPIRO, M.D.

Investigation of the family contribution to pathologic outcome in adolescence suggests that because of his particular emotional meaning to his parents, the adolescent who is disturbed has not been supported by his parents in his efforts to accomplish phase-appropriate life tasks during the course of his development. On the contrary his parents have responded to his development with anxiety and repudiation of change in their relationships with him. In the face of progressive individuation of the child and adolescent, characteristic defensive behaviors are mobilized in these parents which distort their perceptions of the developing child and adolescent and dominate their responses to him. Members of my research group have reported findings from observations of family interaction indicating that borderline, narcissistic, and acting-out character organizations in adolescents are related in highly specific ways to the characteristics of defensive distortions in the relationships between the parents and the developing child and adolescent (Shapiro, 1967, 1968, 1969; Shapiro, Zinner, Shapiro and Berkowitz, 1975; Shapiro and Zinner, 1976; Shapiro, Shapiro, Zinner and Berkowitz, 1977; Zinner and Shapiro, E., 1975; Zinner and Shapiro, R., 1972, 1974; Berkowitz, Shapiro, Zinner and Shapiro, 1974a, 1974b). Further, our evidence suggests that these defensive responses in parents are related to the nature of their unconscious fantasies regarding the child.

We find evidence in these families of an organization of shared or complementary unconscious fantasies and related defenses within family members, which maintain equilibrium among family members. Anxiety and defensive responses are activated by behavior mobilizing underlying assumptions which derive from unconscious fantasies. We conceptualize these as the unconscious assumptions of the family as a group. When repetitive behaviors in families appear to militate against change, development and individuation of the child, we infer shared unconscious assumptions in family members which motivate and organize these behaviors. Unconscious assumptions are assumed to derive from the internalized developmental experience of both of the parents in their families of origin. An organization of motives and defenses evolves, then, in the marriage, which is operative throughout the development of the child and adolescent. Depending upon their centrality and coerciveness as the family develops, unconscious assumptions are powerful determinants of disturbance in the maturing child and adolescent.

In this chapter I will discuss implications of these findings for the treatment of seriously disturbed adolescents and will suggest that treatment of the family concurrent with individual treatment is indicated for borderline, severely narcissistic, and antisocial, acting-out adolescents. Concurrent individual and family treatment is facilitated by the theory of unconscious assumptions. The theory allows an integration of analytic group concepts required for interpretive family therapy and concepts of analytic individual psychology required in individual psychotherapy.

First I will elucidate the theory of unconscious assumptions. Then, with illustrations from a case example, I will discuss the application of this theory to analytic, group-interpretative family therapy.

THE THEORY OF UNCONSCIOUS ASSUMPTIONS

The concept of unconscious assumptions of the family group is a construct which originates in clinical observation. It derives from the small group theory of Bion (1961; Rioch, 1970). Bion's theory is an analytic group theory, in that it is a conceptualiation of both the conscious tasks which define groups and the unconscious motives in group members which may dominate group behavior. Our effort to conceptualize family behavior has been facilitated by using a similar framework, that of family tasks and of a variety of unconscious motives which interfere with their achievement. From the point of view of adolescent development, we conceive of the family as having great importance in promoting specific developmental tasks (Shapiro, 1963, 1967). These include the promotion of relative ego autonomy and an integrated identity formation in adolescent family members leading to their individuation and to a changed emotional relationship to their parents and to peers (Shapiro, 1969; Blos, 1962; Erikson, 1950, 1956). Adolescent development is impaired by unconscious assumptions in the family which militate against the task of adolescent individuation. States of anxiety and defense are activated in the family in response to normal developmental manifestations of this period. Regression and symptomatic behavior are then evident in family members; they are often most marked in the adolescent.

A brief review of Bion's small group theory will help us to clarify its application to family process. In the theory of Bion, a group is defined by the task it is gathered to do. Consciously motivated behavior directly implementing this task in reality terms is called work group functioning. Bion observes that much behavior in groups appears to have some other motivation. This behavior suggest an unconscious assumption on the part of members that the group is gathered for quite different purposes than the realistic accomplishment of the work task. Bion postulates unconscious mechanisms in group members which are mobilized in group interrelationships and which result in behavior unconcerned with the considerations of reality. He designates as basic assumptions these states in groups where behavior appears to be determined by shared wishful, nonrational, unconscious considerations. In such states a group appears to be dominated and often united by covert assumptions based on unconscious fantasies.

Bion outlines three general categories of basic assumptions which he frequently sees dominating the behavior of groups. One is the unconscious assumption that the group exists for satisfaction of dependency needs and wishes (basic assumption *dependency*); another is the assumption that the group exists to promote aggression toward or to provide the means of flight from reality objects, issues, and tasks (basic assumption *fight-flight*); the third is an assumption of hope and an atmosphere of expectation which is unrelated to reality considerations and is frequently seen in relation to pairing behavior in the group (basic assumption *pairing*). The basic assumption mode of group behavior then is formulated from behavior which implies covert and often unconscious assumptions in group members about the purpose for which the group is gathered. Basic assumption group behavior is mobilized for defensive purposes having to do with the difficulties of the work task and disturbance in relation to the work leader. The work of the group—its functioning and its task performance—is impaired with deterioration of the ego functioning of the members. The realities of the situation and the task are lost sight of, reality testing is poor, secondary process thinking deteriorates, and more primitive forms of thinking emerge. There is a new organization of behavior which seems to be determined by fantasies and assumptions which are unrealistic and represent a failed struggle to cope with the current reality situation. The group itself survives, though its essential functioning and primary task are now altered in the service of a different task (Turquet, 1974).

Bion's theory provides a useful framework for organizing clinical observations of the family. States of anxiety, defense and regression in the family are conceptualized as consequences of unconscious assumptions, in which an organization of meanings, motives and defenses is inferred. These assumptions are in opposition to the tasks of the family with respect to the development of its adolescent members. Family group behavior becomes dominated by assumptions that particular meanings of adolescent individuation and autonomy represent a danger to family requirements, cohesiveness and even survival. These assumptions are generally unconscious and may be denied by family members.

The family group is different in essential ways from the small group of strangers as conceptualized by Bion. However, the study of the family is facilitated through observing the shifts from family behavior implementing reality tasks to family behavior dominated by unconscious assumptions. In considering the nuclear family as a group, the fact that its members have both a shared developmental history and specific role relationships results in a differentiation and specificity of shared assumptions, motivations and defenses which cannot exist in the randomness of the stranger group.

In this sense, the complexity and differentiation of family process are much closer to individual psychodynamics than to group process. It is therefore possible to make discriminating analyses of the dynamics of family regression, of specific characteristics of shared unconscious fantasies and assumptions in families, and of the characteristics of shared and complementary defensive behaviors between and among family members. In contrast, formulations about basic assumption behavior in stranger groups are global and generalized conceptualizations of group regression and of regressive group wishes in relation to the leader.

Let us now consider the evidence in family interaction which leads us to infer that unconscious assumptions are dominating family behavior. When the family is in a situation of anxiety as a consequence of mobilization of unconscious assumptions, we find clear analogies to small group basic assumption behavior. Behavior showing conflicting motivations, anxiety, and defense is seen in family members, with frequent evidence of ego regression. Behavior in the family appears to be determined more by fantasy than by reality. Work failure, similar to basic assumption functioning, is evident in the family situation. There is emergence of confused, distorted thinking; failure of understanding and adequate communication; and breakdown in the ability of the family to work cooperatively or creatively in relation to developmental issues and tasks, to maintain a progressive discussion in which family members understand each other, or to deal realistically with the problems under discussion. In short, when the family is in a situation in which unconscious assumptions are mobilized, associated anxiety and a variety of defensive behaviors are seen and there is disturbance in the family's reality functioning. In contrast, in the absence of mobilization of unconscious assumptions, the family does not manifest anxiety and defensive behavior, is clearly reality oriented, and is well related to tasks facilitating the maturation of children and adolescents.

In order to characterize the family contributions to adolescent disturbance, we study carefully episodes of family regression determined by unconscious assumptions. We observe transactions between the parents and adolescent in order to define defensive meanings of these relationships implicit in the behavior. And we infer from these defensive behaviors unconscious meanings of the adolescent to the parents and of the parents to the adolescent, allowing more precise formulations of unconscious assumptions of the family as a group.

We use the concept of delineation to formulate the dynamics of these relationships. Delineations are behaviors through which one family member communicates explicitly or implicitly his perceptions and attitudes—in fact, his mental representation of another family member—to that other person. Delineations may communicate a view of the other person which seems to be predominantly determined by his reality characteristics. Or delineations may communicate a view of the other person which appears to be predominantly determined by the mobilization of dynamic conflict and defense in the delineator. We call the latter category defensive delineations. When delineations are observed to be distorted, stereotyped and over-specific, contradictory, or otherwise incongruent with the range of behaviors manifested by the family member being delineated, we make the inference that these delineations serve a defensive need. That is, they are not simply realistic characterizations of the family member being delineated. And we further hypothesize that through their defensive delineations family members seek to maintain others in relatively fixed roles in the service of avoiding their own anxiety.

The predominant mechanism underlying defensive delineations is projective identification (Zinner and Shapiro, 1972). The concept of projective identification provides a means of conceptualizing phenomena of regression and of elucidating dynamics of role allocation in families. In family regression there is rapid reduction in usual ego discriminations. Dissociation and projection are increased with confusion over the ownership of personal characteristics which are easily attributed to other family members. When one individual assumes a role compatible with the attributions of others in the family at the regressed level, he quickly becomes the recipient of projections which tend to fix him in that role. Family members project this aspect of their own personal characteristics into him and unconsciously identify with him. The power of these projections with their accompanying unconscious identifications may, over time, push the individual into more extreme role behavior.

In families of disturbed adolescents we find conspicuous parental defensive delineations of the adolescent. These parental projections have a critical effect on the individual child and adolescent maturing within the framework of family group assumptions. Identification processes are internalizations which are central determinants of structure formation in the child. In addition, we believe that the child internalizes, throughout his development, aspects of family relationships in which the parents attribute particular characteristics to him and communicate attitudes towards him. These delineations also modify the child's self-representation and are determinants of structure formation. Delineations of the child and adolescents which serve a defensive function for the parent are particularly coercive, in that behavior in the child incongruent with these parental delineations leads to anxiety in the parent. The child is then motivated to behave so as to mitigate this parental anxiety. Internalization by the child of the parent's projections into him moves the developing child and adolescent into a role which is complementary to parental defensive requirements, with which the parent unconsciously identifies. These defensive delineations are consequently dynamic determinants of role allocation in the family. The role allocated is necessary to maintain parental defense and mitigate parental anxiety. The dynamics of role allocation operate in a broader framework of unconscious assumptions of the family as a group. These, over time, establish a pattern of internalizations within the self-representation. Unconscious assumptions within the family and related experiences of projective identification impinge upon the reorganization of internalizations required by ego-id maturation during adolescence. These influences may interfere significantly with individuation and the consolidation of identity in the adolescent.

THE APPLICATION OF THE THEORY OF UNCONSCIOUS ASSUMPTIONS TO ANALYTIC, GROUP-INTERPRETIVE FAMILY THERAPY

In family assessment and family therapy we attempt to articulate the unconscious assumptions of the family as a group and to discern the participation, contribution and collusion of each family member in episodes of family regression dominated by unconscious assumptions.

In interpretive treatment with the family, our guiding formulations are around unconscious assumptions. In the treatment plan we utilized in our research at the National Institute of Mental Health, family therapy was concurrent with individual and marital therapy, with one of the family co-therapists acting as the individual therapist, for the adolescent, and the other family co-therapist acting as the marital therapist for the parents. We were able to deepen our understanding of family group assumptions in the individual and marital therapy sessions. In the family therapy, an interpretive focus on unconscious assumptions allowed clarification of the relation of each family member to the central dynamic issues within the family. Interpretation effected a reduction in projective identification and promoted reinternalization of qualities within individual family members which had been dissociated and projected in episodes of family regression.

A case example will illustrate the data from which we infer family regression determined by unconscious assumptions. It will demonstrate shared characteristics in family members which are the focus of interpretive interventions in family therapy.

Case Report

In this family, a dramatic personality change occurred in the adolescent, a boy of 18, during his first two years of college. This reached a crisis with feelings of confusion, of merging with others, of being controlled by others, with extreme shifts in mood and rage episodes which finally resulted in his hospitalization.

In the hospital we made the diagnosis of bordeline character organization because of evidence of identity diffusion, relatively intact reality testing, and manifestations of splitting of contradictory ego states which seemed to dominate his psychological functioning (Kernberg, 1975). Extreme shifts were seen from ego states which were positive (libidinally cathected), manifested in euphoria and mystical experiences, to ego states which were negative (aggressively cathected), manifested in feelings of unworthiness, rage, and despair; also, he experienced feelings of being extremely vulnerable to the attitudes and to the control of other people.

The parents of the adolescent were extremely concerned about his welfare. They were cooperative about his hospitalization and about their participation in our program. They appeared to be intelligent people, with extremely conventional responses and attitudes. Both stated that they found the adolescent's difficulties incomprehensible.

The father's parents died during his teens and he described a long, difficult period of struggle to support himself and his siblings. The mother remained extremely close to her own mother until the latter's death 10 years previously.

The parents agreed that the adolescent had presented no difficulties until going away to college. They had been pleased at his going to college but would have preferred his attending college in the city in which they lived. However, when a prestigious university in another state accepted him as a student they supported his going there and emphasized their pleasure at his accomplishment and their interest in his growing up and becoming independent.

Observations of interaction in this family revealed a far more complicated set of feelings and attitudes than the parents reported in their initial discussions with us. In actual observations of the family in conjoint therapy, repeated evidences of struggle over independent behavior and functioning of each of the family members were seen. When thinking or action of one family member was perceived as independent of the control of other family members, that person appeared to become frustrating and "bad" in the view of the others and interactions having the aim of repudiation and control were regularly seen. These appeared to be efforts to re-establish a "good" (positive) relationship. Differences were clearly interpreted within the family as attacks. They seemed to imply a serious threat of loss and alienation. This was particularly true when differences and disagreements were expressed by the adolescent. His parents' attitudes toward him communicated their expectation of conformity and their intense antagonism to behavior independent of their supervision. Similar reactions were seen within the family to differences between the parents.

These findings are illustrated by excerpts from tape-recorded family therapy sessions. The first excerpt is taken from a conjoint family session which occurred 10 months after the patient's admission to the hospital. The adolescent has been talking in recent family sessions about returning to college in several months. He has been working successfully for two months outside the hospital at a part-time job. He raises the issue of college again in this session, but this time it is coupled with a new and more immediate project. He states that he wants to leave the hospital as soon as possible, but to move into an apartment of his own rather than live again with his parents.

Excerpt 1

Allen: . . . I'm thinking of leaving here and getting an apartment on the outside . . . and I think I've found that . . . for my *own* good, the approval I want is the absence of disapproval.

Father: That I don't understand. I don't know what the absence of disapproval means.

Mother: Either you approve or you disapprove.

Allen: Well, you don't disapprove or don't approve. You can . . .

Mother: In other words, you're going to do this regardless of how we feel. Is that it?

Father: No, no—that isn't what he's trying to say . . .

Mother: The absence of disapproval . . .

Allen: That's probably true, though, anyway. But that's not what I said. It's *your* interpretation.

Mother: Well, I'm interested in hearing what your plans are.

Father: I mean getting to the point of absence of disapproval— I mean I just don't get it! He—even if we sat and didn't say a word about it, you would *know* whether we approved or disapproved.

Allen: How? . . . How?

Father: I think you lived with us long enough and know our thoughts and our ways and . . .

Allen: (*quickly*) And you—you haven't changed any of them.

Father: Huh? Basically, I don't think so.

Allen: I was afraid of that.

Father: I don't think you've changed any . . . basically either.

Mother: But in order to give you our approval or disapproval, we have to know what it is you're planning. If you go into an apartment . . .

Allen: . . . it's a way of defending myself.

Therapist: Against what?

Father: What are you defending against?

Allen: Against both of you.

Mother: (*rather vehemently*) I want to know that if you go into an apartment that you're going to live like a human being.

Therapist: Which is . . .?

Mother: Which is—knowing that he's going to have three meals a day, because I know how negligent he has been about his meals, even being here . . .

Allen: (low voice) I don't get three meals a day here either.

Mother: Well, that's your own fault! I know that he gets up late and he hasn't been eating breakfast—and he has his lunch, maybe 3 o'clock, maybe not. Then he has no supper! . . . and *that's* under proper supervision. Now what's he going to do if he's in an apartment by himself?

Therapist: You seem to feel he'll need a supervisor.

Mother: (brief pause) Well, that's what I mean! Those things concern me. He's—unless he realizes that these things are important—to his health and his maintenance—he has to know that he's—that he has to go to sleep on time. If he doesn't get enough sleep, which he feels isn't important, at least he didn't—and I had hoped already that he had thought that eating was important. (*This speech spoken with much feeling.*)

Allen: I'm surprised you haven't brought this up earlier. It's the first time you've mentioned this since . . .

Mother: And if he goes into an apartment . . . I mean, when you say "apartment," you can get a one-room apartment, you can get a two-room, three-room apartment . . . I want to know that he's with somebody.

This interaction exempifies the mother's delineation of Allen as someone whose moves toward independence are attacks. She counters with anxiety and rage and with behavior which communicates her unquestioned right to control him. She defends her delineation of him with great energy, insisting that she know Allen's plans in order to register her approval or disapproval. She feels that unless she exerts great force her son will not acquiesce to her. Her response to his move away from her implies that it will threaten his survival.

Her need to control and constrain him appears automatic and unyielding. We take this to be evidence that this delineation serves a defensive purpose for the mother. Allen's efforts to differentiate himself from his mother result in her projecting into him characteristics of destructiveness which are mobilized within her when a symbiotic equilibrium is threatened. We understand these anxieties as deriving from her relationship to her own mother, from whom she could not emotionally separate. She felt starved when her mother died and projects anxieties about survival into her son.

The father delineates Allen as someone who knows what his parents are thinking and who must be controlled by their requirements. He communicates an extremely pessimistic attitude about the possibility for increased independence and for change. The father is unable to differentiate Allen from himself. He projects into Allen his feelings of the inevitability of compliance in the interest of family harmony.

In later family sessions, which followed his discharge from the hospital to live in an apartment of his own, Allen became more overtly attacking and provocative of his parents than they were of him. He became increasingly intolerant of his *mother's* differences from *him* as she was intolerant of his differences from her. He was depressed and anxious living alone and spent many weekends at home. This is a discussion of a weekend at home:

Excerpt 2

Mother: (*Very accusing voice*) And you feel that I'm so . . . ignorant . . . that I'm so moronic—and he told me last night . . . he informed me that I should go to *college!*

Allen: (*Quickly*) I didn't say that.

Mother: Well, that I should educate myself more . . .

Allen: You're not getting along with me very well either. You don't know how to get along with *me* . . .

Mother: No. I don't know how to get along with you at all—you're the only person I can't get along with! Evidently. (*pause*) *And* I'd like to know the reason *why!* Because no matter . . . how much education I would get, you would still be . . . educationwise, above my level *anyway*. And I have no intentions of getting more education just for your sake!

Allen: (*Starts to speak but Father intervenes.*)

Father: This, I think, is a basic . . .

Mother: (*louder*) I don't know *what* it is . . .

Father: I think your—I think your basic thing is—to understand each other better . . . and to try, *try*, to make a point of understanding each other better and do it different ways. Not *one* way.

Mother: *Well*, I think I *try* to understand Allen and I . . . I know that I . . . what he expects of me and what he doesn't want me to say and . . . when I ask him something and if he feels I'm trespassing on his privacy, well, he's very wrong. (*Hurt tone*)

Therapist: Apparently Allen has hurt *you* quite a bit.

Mother: Yes, he has! . . . because for the greater part of the day I mean he's—just like his old self (*Allen:* Old!) but then it seems as though all of a sudden a screw turns—and it's the other side of the record!

The delineations in this excerpt reflect the mother's view of Allen as attacking and controlling *her,* attempting to force her to conform to his requirements. He is now the persecutor who demands that she join his world. Here the father is in the role of mediator between them. The mother sees her son's anger and criticism as implying a demand that she should change. Allen is having great difficulty sustaining a separation from his parents and attempts to repair a separation in which he feels alienated by changing her as she has tried to change him. It is clear in this interaction that these behaviors of Allen generate anxiety in his mother and stimulate her own coercive and controlling behavior.

In later family sessions, the father gradually revealed more of his own thinking and attempted to differentiate himself from the mother. This resulted in a shift away from the old alignments of the father joining the mother in argument against the adolescent, or the father as mediator. Now a new alignment between the father and the adolescent was seen, with the mother again being perceived as controlling and reacting to differences as attacks. Early in a session two months later the father says that he missed Allen when he didn't visit home last weekend. He goes on to amplify his reasons for this.

Excerpt 3

Father: . . . I actually think it was, uh—probably I use him for somebody to lean on.
Therapist: How do you mean?
Father: Well, maybe as somebody that can understand me . . . a lot of times we get into . . . discussion . . . and . . . reasoning and things—he hears me out . . . I think this is important. (*Low voice, slight laugh*) Nobody understands me anymore!
Therapist: "Nobody" being . . .
Father: (*Low voice*) Well, in our family . . . people in our family—that I'm more, so intimate with—you know, the family group. (*Therapist:* Like?) . . . like my wife, like my sister-in-law, like my brother-in-law . . . I guess that's part of it.
Mother: (*Irritated voice*) So I suppose that every time *you* disagree with *me* I'm supposed to say you don't understand me. Is this the idea?
Father: Well, if I disagree with you, I don't *understand* you . . .
Mother: Well . . .
Therapist: So you've been having disagreements all week?

> *Father:* I guess we've been having them, but I guess this past
> week was the ... no more than usual, but the fact that ...
> I feel like I'm ... sort of lost. *(short laugh)*
>
> *Mother:* Nobody's trying to change you! Because you know
> they think a great deal of you! Even though you *think* that
> they don't! *(pause)* Well, elaborate.

> There is a great tension over the father's disagreement with the
> mother. Allen is defined by the father as similar to him and as
> the only one in the family who understands some aspects of
> what he says and thinks. The father makes it explicit that he
> cannot conceive of disagreement if people understand each
> other. He feels lost without the support and agreement of the
> mother, a feeling which has been expressed most frequently by
> Allen.

Let us now specify what unconscious assumptions may be inferred
from these observations of family behavior. Repeated observations
of episodes of anxiety and turmoil in this family lead to formulations about a powerful cluster of unconscious assumptions which
dominate the behavior of the family; they may be stated as follows:

1) Independent thinking and action in family members are
   perceived as destructive attacks and must be thwarted.
2) For this reason control over possible deviance must be exercised constantly.
3) Behaviors implying individuation of family members constitute hostile attacks.
4) Attributes of authority in family members are closely tied
   to fantasies of omniscience and may not be questioned.
5) Independent behavior and thinking contain a grave threat
   of separation and alienation.
6) Massive anxiety is inherent in this threat of separation
   which may lead to personality dissolution or physical
   disorder.

These unconscious assumptions are inferred from repeated examples of family regression in which there is evidence of primitive
splitting in one family member and projection of split-off, "bad"
autonomous aspects of the self into another family member who is
manifesting individuation. From the point of view of the adolescent
ego deficit, independent behaviors on the part of the adolescent regularly produce anxiety in the mother with ego regression, splitting

and projection of rage and destructiveness into the adolescent. The father also manifests anxiety over independent behavior. We suggest that the ego deficit of the adolescent, manifested in impairment in his capacity to integrate split ego states organized around a positive (libidinal) object relationship and a negative (aggressive) object relationship, is derived from repeated experiences throughout his development of parental projection of rage and destructiveness into him when he manifested behavior implying individuation.

The adolescent has matured in a family in which behavior of any family member expressing thinking or action independent of other family members is reacted to as if it were an attack threatening the family with the loss of one of its members. The evidence of repeated episodes of family regression in reaction to independent behavior and separation leads to the inference that shared unconscious assumptions regarding the dangers of these behaviors dominate the family and mobilize primitive defenses of splitting and projection in family members. Interpretive family therapy focuses on these unconscious assumptions. With continued interpretation in the family therapy and related interpretive work in the individual and marital therapy, diminution in the quantity of splitting and projective identification was seen. In the case example, both the adolescent and the father were attempting to differentiate from the mother. This development continued and was less threatening to the mother later in therapy. The case excerpts are selected to emphasize the fundamental consideration that, in our method of family therapy, we attempt to elucidate the participation, contribution and collusion of *each* family member in episodes of family regression dominated by unconscious assumptions.

COMPARISON OF FAMILIES OF DISTURBED ADOLESCENTS

Comparison of families of borderline adolescents, narcissistic adolescents, and antisocial, acting-out adolescents reveals differences in the focus of family unconscious assumptions, and in the nature of defenses in episodes of family regression.

Borderline Adolescents

Parents of borderline adolescents manifest primitive splitting and projection of "badness" as the dominant mechanisms underlying defensive delineations of the adolescent (Shapiro et al., 1975; Shapiro et al., 1977; Zinner and Shapiro, 1975). We find evidence of a range of unconscious assumptions leading to defensive splitting and projection in these families. In certain of these families, dependency needs of the child are perceived as destructive and the phase-appropriate needs of the adolescent for affection and care are then repudiated by both parents and adolescent. In other families the child is fundamentally perceived as a gratifier of parental symbiotic needs; both parents and adolescent respond with great anxiety to phase-appropriate requirements for individuation and separation. On this basis, assumptions of compliance and sameness are required of family members, with the family boundary then containing what is good and the bad being projected outside the family. If the adolescent differentiates himself from other family members in his expression of needs and impulses or ideas, he is perceived as destructive and suffers feelings of extreme alienation from other family members.

Narcissistic Adolescents

Parents of narcissistic adolescents show narcissistic vulnerability, manifested in extreme vacillations between contradictory states of self-regard and overdependence on the confirming approval of external objects, which parallels these characteristics in the adolescent himself (Berkowitz et al., 1974a, 1974b). The unconscious assumptions of these families recruit the child as a narcissistic object whose basic function is perceived as maintaining parental self-esteem by colluding in reenacting with the parents significant relationships that affected the parents' self-esteem in their families of origin. The parents experience phase-appropriate separation-individuation of the adolescent as a narcissistic loss and injury, and regress to a mode of relationship that is increasingly dominated by projection as behaviors of adolescent that herald separation and autonomy threaten precarious parental self-esteem. In their resulting narcissistic rage, the parents often reactively devalue the adolescent and attempt to restore their own narcissistic equilibrium by projecting onto him their disowned, negative valuations of themselves. In the adolescent, parental rage precipitates a narcissistic regression to fixations which originated in childhood struggles over separation-individuation.

Antisocial Adolescents

Parents of antisocial, acting-out adolescents are more differentiated than the parents of borderline adolescents (Zinner and Shapiro, 1974). Projective mechanisms are the basis of defensive delineations, but the projections are less massive and are likely to be differentiated aspects of impulse life like particular forms of sexual behavior (e.g., promiscuity, homosexuality), with more differentiated superego responses being retained within the parents. Unconscious assumptions are relatively differentiated fantasies which contain anxieties and concerns of the parents rising from their own internal conflicts, with one element in the conflict being projected onto the developing adolescent. These unconscious fantasies differ from family to family but contain in them fantasies originating in one or both parents (e.g., fantasies of promiscuity, homosexual fantasies, etc.), which are projected by the parents onto the adolescent. Covert gratification of these impulses in the parent or parents then occurs through their identification with the adolescent.

INDICATIONS FOR FAMILY THERAPY

The more severe disturbances of adolescence—the borderline conditions, severe narcissistic pathology, and antisocial acting-out—present a specific indication for ongoing treatment of the family, concurrent with individual psychotherapy of the adolescent, because of the severe pathology in the family over separation-individuation.

Moreover, adequate assessment of any adolescent patient includes assessment of the family in addition to interviews with the adolescent alone. In family interviews, assessment of the external resistances to treatment must be accomplished, i.e., assessment of the nature of the adolescent's dependency on his parents and the nature of resistances in the family to change in the adolescent. In addition to their value for assessment of external resistances, conjoint family interviews have the goal of forming a beginning working alliance with the parents, as well as with the adolescent. It is important that this alliance be established and general goals of treatment agreed upon. Family interviews during the assessment phase establish a working situation which can be held in reserve and, in the most favorable cases, may not be needed again (Shapiro, 1978).

If, however, the disturbance in the adolescent is related to conflict between members of the family, change in the adolescent may
give rise to external resistances on the part of the parents. This
possibility should be anticipated in the assessment phase. A recon-
vening of family interviews is then indicated to attempt to manage
the external resistances through interpretive work with the family.
In conjoint family interviews, exploration of the nature and source
of the impasse between parents and adolescent is possible. The therapist is aided in his effort to maintain a stance of neutrality by
orienting himself to the goals of therapy the family has agreed upon
and proceeding with the task of examining interferences with the
accomplishment of these goals. The framework of family interviews established during the assessment phase is the situation which
authorizes the therapist to work interpretively on this task. He attempts to understand and interpret the resistances in the family to
change in the adolescent, both from the side of the parents and
the side of the adolescent. The psychotherapy of adolescents with
severe neuroses or higher order character pathology may then be
preserved through analysis of resistances in the family to change in
the adolescent.

SUMMARY

This chapter has presented some concepts we have found useful in
the treatment of families of disturbed adolescents. We find in these
families an organization of shared or complementary unconscious
fantasies and related defenses within family members which maintain equilibrium in the family group. Unconscious assumptions of
the family as a group are evidenced in repetitive behaviors in families which appear to militate against change, development or individuation of children and adolescents. Shared unconscious assumptions in family members which motivate and organize these repetitive behaviors derive from the internalized developmental experience of both of the parents in their families of origin. An organization of motives and defenses evolves, then, in the marriage. These
shared unconscious assumptions are operative throughout the development of the children and adolescents and have critical effects
on their personality development. Depending upon their centrality
and coerciveness as the family develops, unconscious assumptions

are powerful determinants of disturbance in the maturing children and adolescents. From the theory of unconscious assumptions we generate the central formulations utilized in analytic, group-interpretive treatment of families.

In the treatment of adolescents, unconscious assumptions in the family may lead to resistances in the family to change in the adolescent. Conjoint family interviews during the assessment phase establish a working alliance with the family which can be utilized in the management of these external resistances.

For neurotic adolescents, conjoint family interviews should be resumed when the external resistances become a serious interference with treatment.

For adolescents manifesting borderline, narcissistic or antisocial, acting-out character pathology, where serious disturbances over separation-individuation are found in both adolescents and parents, concurrent interpretive family therapy and individual psychotherapy for the adolescent are indicated.

REFERENCES

BERKOWITZ, D., SHAPIRO, R., ZINNER, J., & SHAPIRO, E. Family contributions to narcissistic disturbances in adolescents. *Int. Rev. Psychoanal.*, 1:353-362, 1974. (a)

BERKOWITZ, D., SHAPIRO, R., ZINNER, J., & SHAPIRO, E. Concurrent family treatment of narcissistic disorders in adolescents. *Int. J. Psychoanal. Psychother.*, 3:399-411, 1974. (b)

BION, W. R. *Experiences in Groups*. London: Tavistock Publications, 1961.

BLOS, P. *On Adolescence: A Psychoanalytic Interpretation*. New York: The Free Press of Glencoe, 1962.

ERIKSON, E. *Childhood and Society*. New York: Norton, 1950.

ERIKSON, E. The problem of ego identity. *J. Amer. Psychoanal. Assoc.*, 4:56-121, 1956.

KERNBERG, O. *Borderline Conditions and Pathological Narcissism*. New York: Aronson, 1975.

RIOCH, M. The work of Wilfred Bion on groups. *Psychiatry*, 33:56-66, 1970.

SHAPIRO, E., ZINNER, J., SHAPIRO, R., & BERKOWITZ, D. The influence of family experience on borderline personality development. *Int. Rev. Psychoanal.* 2(4):399-411, 1975.

SHAPIRO, E., SHAPIRO, R., ZINNER, J., & BERKOWITZ, D. The borderline ego and the working alliance: Indications for family and individual treatment in adolescence. *Int. J. Psychoanal.*, 58(1):77-89, 1977.

SHAPIRO, R. Adolescence and the psychology of the ego. *Psychiatry*, 26:77-87, 1963.

SHAPIRO, R. The origin of adolescent disturbances in the family: Some considerations in theory and implications for therapy. In G. Zuk & I. Boszormenyi-Nagy (Eds.), *Family Therapy and Disturbed Families*. Palo Alto: Science and Behavior Books, 1967.

SHAPIRO, R. Action and family interaction in adolescence. In J. Marmor (Ed.), *Modern Psychoanalysis*. New York: Basic Books, 1968.

SHAPIRO, R. Adolescent ego autonomy and the family. In G. Caplan & S. Lebovici (Eds.), *Adolescence: Psychosocial Perspectives*. New York: Basic Books, 1969.

SHAPIRO, R. & ZINNER, J. Family organization and adolescent development. In E. Miller (Ed.), *Task and Organization*. London; New York: John Wiley and Sons, 1976, pp. 289-308.

SHAPIRO, R. The adolescent, the therapist, and the family: The management of external resistances to the psychoanalytic therapy of adolescents. *J. Adolescence*, 1:1-8, 1978.

TURQUET, P. Leadership, the individual and the group. In Gibbard G. S., Hartman, J. J., & Mann, R. D. (Eds.), *Analysis of Groups*. San Francisco: Jossey-Bass, 1974.

ZINNER, J. & SHAPIRO, R. Projective identification as a mode of perception and behavior in families of adolescents. *Int. J. Psychoanal.*, 53:523-529, 1972.

ZINNER, J. & SHAPIRO, R. The family group as a single psychic entity: Implications for acting out in adolescence. *Int. Rev. Psychoanal.*, 1:179-186, 1974.

ZINNER, J. & SHAPIRO, E. Splitting in families of borderline adolescents. In J. Mack (Ed.), *Borderline States in Psychiatry*. New York: Grune and Stratton, 1975, pp. 103-122.

12

Use of Psychotropic Medication in Adolescent Psychiatry

DONALD McKNEW, JR., M.D.

Reviewing psychopharmacology as it applies to adolescents is difficult in a short chapter for reasons that are central to the problem of understanding the subject under discussion. Although it is increasingly apparent that adolescents can benefit from a variety of medications, adolescent drug therapy still remains a very murky and uncharted field. Most clinicians agree that, but for the exceptions that will be mentioned, adolescents benefit from the same psychotropic drugs that benefit adults and that these drugs are, in general, used in the same manner. On the one hand, this makes understanding pharmacology in this area much easier because one merely needs to apply the knowledge about drugs in adults to this group of patients. However, complications arise when one realizes the rapidity with which drug therapy is changing at the current time. New drugs are being discovered and new applications for old drugs are being found, so that one has to constantly be studying in order to stay abreast of this field.

This chapter will first review the only condition that is unique to adolescents in terms of pharmacological therapy; *anorexia nervosa*. Later sections of the chapter will review other drugs that are used with adolescents and some of what is currently known of their psychopharmacology.

DRUG THERAPY IN ANOREXIA NERVOSA

Anorexia nervosa has been extensively studied over the last several years, with Hilda Bruch (1973) making many of the first contributions. In recent years there has been an effort to try to substitute behavioral or drug therapies for more traditional dynamic therapy in the treatment of this puzzling and difficult disorder. The first drug to be used effectively was chlorpromazine. Dally and Sargant (1960) compared chlorpromazine treatment of 20 anorexics with 24 patients treated with other therapies. The chlorpromazine group gained 2 kilograms per week in weight and required an average hospital stay of 34 days, whereas the other group gained little and required 58 days of hospitalization. Chlorpromazine was given in the range of 150 mg to 1000 mg.

The next drug to receive attention was amitriptyline. There was a study reported by Paykel, Mueller and de la Vergne (1973) which showed a mean weight gain of 2.5 kg. over a treatment period as compared to .2 kg. for the patients on placebo.

The most recent drug to be tried in this area is cyproheptadine, which is well-known for its effectiveness in stimulating weight gain and for its paucity of side effects. Goldberg et al. (1977) has reported some preliminary analyses of a study done with 81 anorexia nervosa patients given this drug in a variety of combinations with behavioral modifications. In this study the drug was found to be effective in a subgroup of anorexics who had a history of birth delivery complications, were especially emaciated on entering the study, and had a history of prior outpatient treatment failure. Thus, one finds three drugs of totally different pharmacology all helpful in this syndrome.

DEPRESSION

The clinical syndrome of depression is seemingly a syndrome of catecholamine metabolism dysfunction although, as with most neurochemistry, the final truth is far from clear. This syndrome, which is increasingly evident in adolescents, is very responsive to either the tricyclics, the monoamine oxidase (MAO) inhibitors, or lithium, when these drugs are used appropriately. Because of the importance of the neurochemistry to understanding how one uses these drugs clinically, it will be reviewed first.

Review of Neurochemistry

It has been cited frequently that the tricyclic antidepressants primarily block the reuptake of catecholamines from the synaptic cleft. More recently (U'Prichard et al., 1978), it has also been shown that the alpha noradrenergic receptors have a greater affinity for binding to tertiary amine tricyclics (amitriptyline) than secondary ones (imipramine), leading to the tertiary amines causing more sedation and relieving more psychomotor agitation than the secondary ones, probably through the blocking of serotonin at alpha sites. There is another group of antidepressants that are becoming more commonly used—the MAO inhibitors such as Parnate. This group of drugs specifically inhibits the MAO enzymes that circulate through the cytoplasm near the vesicles that release catecholamines. When these MAO enzymes are allowed to operate, they break down the catecholamines as they return to be taken back up by one of the vesicles. In that case that particular catecholamine is lost for future use. However, with the MAO inhibitors, more catecholamine is taken back into the vesicle and more is available.

When the catecholamines are broken down they form an end product called 3-methoxy-4-hydroxyphenylene glycol (MHPG) which is excreted in the urine and can be easily measured. It is also the only breakdown product that crosses the blood-brain barrier in quantity. For many years it has been known that in most patients, MHPG is decreased in depression and elevated in mania. However, Schildkraut et al. (1973) has shown that there are certain depressive states where MHPG is elevated. He made the discovery that if one gave people with elevated MHPG levels amitriptyline, they improved, while those with lowered MHPG levels improved on imipramine. This is the first time a truly rational way of deciding which of the major antidepressants to use has been available. In addition, recently it has been discovered that the MAO inhibitors can be used quite safely in conjuction with the tricyclic antidepressants. Many especially obsessional, depressed patients will respond quite well to a combination of a tricyclic and an MAO inhibitor.

It has most recently been found that dibenzepine can be given in a 24-hour/day i.v. drip (Saletu et al., 1978). This treatment generally must be continued for two days intravenously followed by three weeks by mouth; the patient frequently recovers from his affective disorder during the first six days. Suffice it to say that very large amounts of medication are given during this period of time. This particular agent is not available in this country at this time, but that situation should be changed in the near future.

Administering Antidepressants

Clinical experience shows that the administration of these medications to adolescents presents few problems. The tricyclics can be effective in very small doses or in very large ones, depending upon the patient. This is apparently due to the degree to which the chemicals pass from the gastrointestinal tract into the bloodstream. Most patients experience a therapeutic effect on the same amount of tricyclic in their bloodstream (Wharton, 1978). If clinical laboratories enjoyed the facilities available in research laboratories, i.e. a method of measuring blood levels of tricyclics, clinicians could prescribe tricyclics with the same scientific accuracy with which they prescribe lithium today, that is, give the medication until it reaches the proper level in the bloodstream. Unfortunately, most clinical laboratories do not supply this information and so the psychiatrist must try moving up and down the scale until he finds that level which is most helpful and where the side effects are not too troublesome. The clinician must be aware that if he begins with the traditional dose of 100 mg/day, it is quite possible that he may have to decrease it rather than increase it.

Most adolescent patients tolerate the side effects of antidepressants fairly well, although the drowsiness at times can be very annoying to more obsessional adolescents. The dry-mouth and other anticholinergic effects can be handled well by the use of urecholine 10-40 mg/day. The usual precautions with MAO inhibitors should be followed, but the MAO inhibitors are not the frightening drugs that we used to think they were. Of course, one drawback of the major antidepressants in youngsters is that they do take a period of time to gain full effectiveness. The effects of imipramine and the MAO inhibitors are more delayed than the effects of amitriptyline. Since adolescents are notoriously impatient, warding off this impatience may be the most difficult task for the psychiatrist. Experience has shown that the drug should be administered for at least six months if a serious depression is present. Wharton (1978) views this as a kind of cellular learning experience that is very important and quite likely to prevent a precipitous recurrence of the affective disorder.

Lithium

Lithium is one of the amazing stories in the recent history of psychiatry. The antimanic effect of lithium was discovered by Cade in Australia in 1945. It was not until some ten years later that a number of psychiatrists began to investigate the properties of this drug in this country. The mechanism of lithium is not clear at this writing. There is evidence that lithium does affect catecholamine metabolism (Schildkraut et al., 1966, 1978) ; it is also known to affect the transport of ions across cell membranes. There has been speculation that lithium may affect the cyclic-AMP system (Corrodi et al., 1967). However, all of these are speculations and no sure answer is available.

Once an adolescent has been diagnosed as unipolar or bipolar affectively disturbed, he should be given the benefit of lithium at least on a trial basis. There are quite startling results with youngsters as young as 13 years of age who have had their whole lives altered through the use of this chemical. It is possible that as many as 30% of the children of manic-depressive adults may have the disease (McKnew et al., in press). The disease expresses itself in many ways. It can appear directly in the form of a manic episode or a severe depression, or it may present itself as a cyclothymic personality, a schizo-affective personality or, at times, as an antisocial personality.

In virtually all of these instances, lithium may be helpful. Lithium should be given in its full therapeutic dose fairly quickly. In the past there was a tendency toward excessive caution, but this is not entirely necessary because one can be guided clearly by the effects. Once the clinician has decided to use lithium, he should start lithium at 300 mg and add until a therapeutic blood level is reached (0.8-1.2 mEq/litre). I always suggest a blood test in three days, followed by adjustments of medication. In three days the full effect of the current dose on the blood level is reached. As soon as the therapeutic blood level is obtained, one should continue medication for at least six months before assuming that the medication is not working. Lithium usually shows its first effect between 6-10 days. This beneficial effect usually continues to manifest itself and grow stronger, with a significant jump in efficacy occurring at nine months.

If lithium is effective it may be needed for life. Since that is the case, it is reasonable at some period, such as after a year, to have a trial without the medication, a "drug vacation," to make sure that there is not a basic placebo effect in operation. Lithium alone is usually most beneficial in bipolar affectively disturbed patients. In unipolar patients, lithium is felt to act more in a prophylactic manner than a therapeutic one. One should usually add a small dose of a tricyclic to the lithium with unipolar patients. The dose of the tricyclic can be as small as 5 or 10 mg. two or three times per day, and still have a beneficial effect when it is combined with the lithium because of the synergistic effect.

MINOR TRANQUILIZERS

The minor tranquilizers we can discuss very briefly. Their exact mode of action is still a matter of controversy. Much of the early research showed the minor tranquilizers working in the substantia-nigra to inhibit dopamine release (Tsuchiga and Fukushima, 1977). More recent work has shown that the minor tranquilizers can be found at almost every site where a GABA neuron terminates (Kozhechkin and Ostrovskaya, 1977). Here these drugs seem to be working in a synergistic manner with the GABA.

However, whatever the mechanism of action of these drugs, they are of little use among adolescents. This is one of the instances where adolescent psychiatry breaks away from adult psychiatric usage. The problem is one of addiction. Adolescents are so prone to abuse these drugs and even use many of these drugs on their own for pleasure, that it is very difficult and usually inadvisable to use them with teenagers except under most unusual circumstances. I think that in school phobias and in certain other anxiety situations it is possible that, with strict supervision, these drugs can be fruitful, but their use in all other situations should be looked on with a jaundiced eye.

Major tranquilizers, on the other hand, are used with adolescents exactly as they are with adults, i.e. for schizophrenia and other psychotic states. The neurochemistry of the phenothiazines and of haloperidol involves the blockade of post-synaptic dopamine receptors. The dopamine hypothesis of schizophrenia states, that in this disorder there is, for unknown reasons, excess dopamine and excess specific receptors. An ancillary hypothesis speculates that the excess dopamine comes from a deficiency of dopamine-β-hydroxylase. If these theories are correct, they would explain why dopamine receptor blockade works in these serious disorders and why it is also extremely helpful to give it to youngsters who have taken certain hallucinogenic drugs. At any rate, schizophrenic disorders seen in adolescence respond well to phenothiazines.

The administration of the phenothiazines and their effects have been presented so amply (Davis, 1975) that little can be added. However, there are a few observations that may be helpful. I have been impressed that rapid administration of one of the phenothiazines can prevent hospitalization or other type of care away from the home. I think therapists are much too timid in their administration of these drugs. It is possible to keep a psychotic, uncontrollable patient in a waiting room or clinic and administer a dose of phenothiazine every hour until the patient is heavily sedated. At that time the family can handle him quite easily. Often, after two or three days of visiting the clinic, the patient is feeling more comfortable and is able to remain out of an institutional setting. It is often the timid use of the phenothiazines that makes for too much hospital care. Of course, that situation is also promoted by many parents becoming discouraged and wanting the children out of their homes.

The psychiatrist may encounter a good deal of resistance from the adolescents who receive phenothiazines, much in the manner as with the tricyclic antidepressants. They object to the drowsiness, they object to the lost control, and they object to the physical alterations in their bodies, such as the dry mouth or blurred vision, which they see as a dangerous and insidious poisoning. Patience, a clear understanding of the side effects and an ample explanation to the youngster are often all that are needed to ward off many battles over these drugs. However, the clinician must be ever mindful that these youngsters can hide the medication, flush it down toilets, throw it away in the street, so that all the while the psychiatrist believes he has a fully medicated youngster on his hands, he has a teenager who is taking no medication at all. It is vital to explain the side effects, to explain the benefits, and to create a cooperative relationship with the youngster. Often, if they see their doctor as trying to keep them out of the hospital, a strong alliance can be formed.

These drugs are extremely safe and can be given in very large doses. They should be given until symptoms have truly abated; the medication can then be reduced to a stable level which should be maintained, once again for approximately nine months. There have been numerous studies (Stevens, 1970) which have all shown that if the phenothiazines are not continued well past the abatement of the original symptoms, there is a much greater chance for a rapid recurrence.

HYPERACTIVITY

The only major group of drugs that have not been discussed are those used for hyperactive adolescents. Extensive research in recent years has shown that hyperactivity is not merely a disorder of childhood but may continue into adulthood. Wood et al. (1976) have even shown that there are some patients in whom the condition is not discovered until adulthood and that these people respond quite as well to Ritalin or Dexedrine as children. Thus, the psychiatrist may find adolescents who represent the classical hyperactive syndrome. In these cases, he should consider Ritalin or Dexedrine. Ritalin does seem to be the preferred drug at the current time. There are some instances where Mellaril also seems to be extremely effective.

SEDATIVES AND SLEEP MEDICATION

Basically, these drugs should not be used with adolescents for the same reason that the minor tranquilizers should not be used. There is a danger of addiction. Once again, these drugs are used widely by adolescents on their own because of the kicks that they get from them. Psychiatrists certainly should not add to their supply of these medications. However, there are some few emergent situations where, with close monitoring, it would seem reasonable to use a sedative medication for a few nights to help the youngster.

SUMMARY

In summary, the psychopharmacology of adolescents is very similar to that of adults. It is primarily in management areas that differences arise. Adolescents may be both more resistant to medication and more likely to abuse it. The field of psychopharmacology is rapidly changing and psychiatrists administering drugs to children, adolescents or adults must keep up with the new and exiciting knowledge available.

REFERENCES

BRUCH, H. *Eating Disorders.* New York: Basic Books, Inc., 1973.

CORRODI, H., FUXE, L., HOKFELT, T., ET AL. Effect of lithium on cerebral monoamine neurons. *Psychopharmacologia*, 11:345-353, 1967.

DALLY, P. J. & SARGANT, W. A new treatment of anorexia nervosa. *Brit. Med. J.*, 1: 1770-1773, 1960.

DAVIS, J. M. Overview: Maintenance therapy in psychiatry: I. Schizophrenics. *Amer. J. Psychiatry*, 132:1237-1245, 1975.

DAVIS, J. M. & COLE, J. O. Antipsychotics. In A. Freedman, H. Kaplan, & B. Sadock (Eds.), *Comprehensive Textbook of Psychiatry*, Vol. II. Baltimore: Williams and Wilkins, 1975.

GOLDBERG, S. C., ECKERT, E., HALMI, K. A., ET AL. Double blind peractin hospital study in anorexia. Read at the annual meeting of the American Psychiatric Association, Toronto, Canada, May 2-6, 1977.

KOZHECHKIN, S. N. & OSTROVSKAYA, R. U. Are benzodiazepines GABA antagonists? *Nature*, 269:72, 1977.

McKNEW, D. H., CYTRYN, L., EFRON, A., ET AL. Offspring of patients with affective disorders. *Brit. J. Psychiatry*, in press.

PAYKEL, E. S., MUELLER, P. S., & DE LA VERGNE, P. M. Amitriptyline, weight gain and carbohydrate craving: A side effect. *Brit. J. Psychiatry*, 123:501-507, 1973.

SALETU, B., STROBL, G., GRUNBERGER, J., ET AL. Intensive antidepressive therapy by 24 hour slow-drip infusion with high doses dibenzepine. *Progr. Neuropsychopharmacol.*, 1:125-134, 1978.

SCHILDKRAUT, J. J. The effects of lithium on norepinephrine turnover and metabolism: Basic and clinical studies. *J. Nerv. Ment. Dis.*, in press.

SCHILDKRAUT, J. J., KEELER, B. A., GRAB, E. L., ET AL. MHPG excretion and clinical classification in depressive disorders. *Lancet*, 1:1251-1252, 1973.
SCHILDKRAUT, J. J., SCHANBERG, S., & KOPIN, I. The effect of lithium ion on H^3 norepinephrine metabolism in brain. *Life Sci.*, 5:1479-1483, 1966.
Schizophrenia Bulletin, Vol. 2, No. 1, 1976.
STEVENS, J. H. Long-term course and prognosis in schizophrenia. *Seminars in Psychiatry*, 2:464-485, 1970.
TSUCHIGA, T. & FUKUSHIMA, H. Effects of benzodiazepines on PGO firings and multiple unit activity in the midbrain reticula formation in cats. *Electroencephalogr. Clin. Neurophysiol.*, 43:700-706, 1977.
U'PRICHARD, D., GREENBERG, D., SHEEHAN, P., ET AL. Tricyclic antidepressants: Therapeutic properties and affinity for alpha-noradrenergic receptor binding sites in the brain. *Science*, 199:197-199, 1978.
WHARTON, R. Personal communication, 1978.
WOOD, D., REIMHERR, F., WENDER, P., ET AL. Diagnosis and treatment of minimal brain dysfunction in adults. *Arch. Gen. Psychiatry*, 33:1453-1460, 1976.

13

Day Hospital Treatment of Adolescents

JOSEPH R. NOVELLO, M.D.

Day hospital programs for adolescents offer several distinct advantages over the more restictive 24-hour (inpatient) hospital programs, on the hand, and traditional outpatient treatment, on the other; yet the day hospital remains the most underutilized resource in all of adolescent psychiatry.

THE CONCEPT OF DAY HOSPITAL

Part of the reason for this underutilization of the day hospital is in widespread confusion among the public, interested "third parties," and even among adolescent psychiatrists themselves as to the very nature and concept of this type of program. The day hospital is not *day care,* which, at best, implies a custodial level of treatment with limited goals of maintaining chronically ill patients at a minimum level of functioning in the community. At worse, *day care,* in the public's mind, usually implies a kind of quasi-sophisticated baby-sitting service.

The day hospital is not a *therapeutic school.* Unfortunately, adolescent day hospital programs, because they normally contain an educational component, are often confused with "special" or therapeutic schools. Such bona fide "school" programs are staffed not by clinicians but by teachers who are skilled in educating emotionally handicapped teenagers. When such "school" programs provide "counseling" or even some ongoing "work" with the students' fam-

215

ilies, confusion with a psychiatric facility is invited. Such programs, of course, either are funded by local school systems or charge private tuitions. They are not medical facilities and are not, therefore, reimbursed by medical insurance carriers.

The day hospital is obviously not a *24-hour hospital*. It is less restrictive than inpatient care, since its patients attend only during the daytime hours while residing at home. At the same time, however, the day hospital is not *outpatient treatment*. It provides for a much more intensive and structured program.

The day hospital is a specific level of psychiatric treatment, quite distinct from each of the four services noted above. Enthusiasts of the concept point out that, for the properly selected adolescent patient, the day hospital can be the best of all possible therapeutic worlds, i.e., it can offer more structure and intensity than just outpatient treatment (or even outpatient treatment in combination with a therapeutic school), without the restrictive and sometimes regressive features of a 24-hour hospital program. Adolescents can avoid a certain amount of possible stigma that is sometimes attached to being hospitalized and parents (and their insurance companies or other funding agencies) can, additionally, benefit from a built-in "cost benefit" factor, since day hospital rates, in general, average only 25-40% of the cost of 24-hour programs.

The day hospital, then, is a true *partial hospitalization program*. It utilizes all of the existing resources of the psychiatric hospital— except the beds. For adolescents, it should contain a well-conceived educational component and a number of other features to be described later in this chapter. Although such programs may also be referred to as "day treatment" (particularly if the facility is "freestanding," i.e., not based at a parent hospital), it should be clear that they are conceived on a medical/psychiatric model and that they treat patients, not students, clients, or "problem kids."

This chapter will describe the basic ingredients of a full day (8:00 a.m. to 5:00 p.m.) program which is a highly structured integration of three basic elements: the partial hospitalization program per se, the therapeutic school program, and the psychotherapy program. Such a comprehensive day hospital program for adolescents is the highest level of partial hospitalization treatment and is designed to accommodate the most seriously disturbed adolescents.

There are other "day treatment" models which can also be employed successfully: a) One is the "evening" or "after school" program for teenagers who are able to attend community schools but require intensive treatment above and beyond traditional outpatient treatment; such programs may operate daily from 4:00 p.m. to 7:00 p.m. or on a more flexible two- or three-day-per-week basis. b) The "weekend" program may offer teenagers treatment and structure on Saturdays and/or Sundays; this type of program is especially suited for adolescents who may be withdrawn and isolated or who tend to decompensate during the relatively unstructured weekend period when, perhaps, intrafamilial conflicts and/or negative peer pressures are especially troublesome.

PURPOSE OF THE DAY HOSPITAL

A clear understanding by all involved of the purpose of the adolescent day hospital program is essential: 1) Is it to be used as an *alternative* to the hospital for certain teenage patients? 2) Is it to be used to *shorten* the hospital stays of adolescents who are already hospitalized? 3) Is it to be used as a short *transition* back to the community for adolescents who have largely completed their treatment while inpatients but who could use a short transitional place to help cushion their reentry to home and community living? 4) Or, finally, is the day hospital to be used for comprehensive, extended evaluations that generally cannot be completed in the usual outpatient programs and would be referred to an evaluation unit of the hospital were it not for the existence of the day hospital?

These four basic uses of the adolescent day hospital are not mutually exclusive. Yet, careful thought must be given to the basic purpose of the program. The purpose will shape the philosophy and will have profound impact on the selection of patients, length of stay, selection of staff and staffing organization, basic program design, the fundamental relationship (or lack of it) with the parent hospital and the school program, the relationship of the program to the community at large, patient and parental acceptance, staff morale, treatment outcome, costs, and reimbursement patterns, as well as on whether the program is called "day hospital," "day treatment," or something else.

The common denominator of the four basic programming philosophies is that the day hospital exists to keep adolescents out of 24-hour hospitals. This is a worthy, but very difficult, goal. Nevertheless, workers in this field generally feel that the day hospital is at its finest when it is designed to treat seriously disturbed adolescents who otherwise would have been directly admitted to the hospital ("alternative" program) and/or hospitalized teenagers who can be discharged more quickly because such an intensive, highly structured program is available ("shorten stays" program). If the program is designed and staffed to treat adolescents in these two groups, it should be able to absorb an occasional patient from group three ("transitional" program) or group four ("evaluation" program).

One word about the 24-hour psychiatric hospital for adolescents: It is *indispensable*. It is indispensable to the disturbed patients whom it treats, for no day hospital program can replace it in the treatment of uncontrollably impulsive adolescents or of adolescents with co-existent serious medical problems. It is also indispensable to the day hospital itself for, if the day program attempts to serve as an "alternative" for some severely disturbed patients, it must have immediate backup from the hospital in the event that a patient requires hospitalization at some point in his treatment course. More will be said later in this chapter on the subject of the many levels of relationships existing between the parent hospital and day hospital programs.

PROGRAM DESCRIPTION

Most day hospitals are physically located within a parent psychiatric facility. Such "hospital-based" programs have the advantages of accessible facilities, availability of staff support, more reliable referral patters from the hospital itself and a firmer medical or psychiatric identity,. Other programs may be located out in the community in office buildings, renovated homes or modified former school buildings. These programs suffer the obvious disadvantages and may not be able to accept some of the more disturbed adolescents that a hospital-based program can accept, but they often are more acceptable to the adolescents themselves and their families; such free-standing programs may also enjoy more staff cohesion, particularly when the staff is firmly identified with the concept of day hospital and prides itself on its independence from a parent organization. Perhaps the best physical arrangement is for the day hospital to be based in its own separate building on the hospital grounds.

Whether the program is hospital-based or free-standing or somewhere in-between, there are three major components to the adolescent day hospital: 1) the partial hospitalization per se or facility component; 2) the school component; 3) the psychotherapy or professional services component. Each of these may be funded by separate sources: partial hospitalization facility charges by hospital insurance, such as Blue Cross, etc.; school tuition by school jurisdictions; and psychotherapy by medical insurance which covers physicians' services, such as Blue Shield.

The Partial Hospitalization Component

The partial hospitalization services and facilities are the very core and essence of the program, making a day hospital truly distinct from intensive outpatient therapy and therapeutic schools.

Medical Model. The day hospital operates on a medical model. Its Director is a child psychiatrist or a general psychiatrist with a particular interest and experience in adolescent psychiatry. He provides overall administrative and clinical supervision of the total program. In addition, the program should have on-site pediatric or medical consultation capability and medical laboratory services. The director may delegate certain day-to-day administrative responsibilities to a Program Administrator, who is usually a psychiatric nurse but who may be a psychologist or psychiatric social worker. A varying number of additional psychiatrists and other mental health professionals are engaged in the clinical treatment of the patients. A senior psychiatric consultant is a most desirable assistant, both as clinical consultant to the staff and as clinical/administrative consultant to the director.

Psychiatric Nursing. Psychiatric nurses may serve in both administrative and clinical roles under the supervision of the psychiatrist. They, in turn, supervise the staff of psychiatric technicians who generally serve to monitor patient behavior and rule compliance and to maintain the behavior modification program when one exists.

The role of psychiatric nurses in an adolescent day hospital could be the subject of a separate chapter, as their function may be substantially different from that of their inpatient colleagues. In addition to handling customary administrative and clinical duties (including medication-giving), they must relate to a host of individuals outside the program, including school personnel, probation officers, referring psychiatrists, etc.; they must also maintain the philosophy of a program that often runs counter to their hospital-based education in nursing school.

Medical Records. Record-keeping in the day hospital generally follows procedures established for the inpatient programs and includes such essentials as admission history and physical, basic laboratory data (including complete blood count, biochemical profile, serology urinalysis and chest x-ray), nursing interview, family interview, initial treatment plan, regular progress, notes, doctor's orders, and discharge summary. As more psychiatric hospitals adopt the Problem-Oriented Record, day hospitals follow suit.

Medical Review. The day hospital must meet specific standards for ambulatory psychiatric facilities established by the Joint Commission on Accreditation of Hospitals (JCAH) and other accrediting agencies. These standards apply to a wide variety of features, including physical facilities, staffing pattern, record-keeping, etc. In addition, the program is subject to review by interested third parties, including Peer Standard Review Organizations (PSRO) and insurance companies. The program may also undergo internal scrutiny by committees for quality assurance, medical audit, medical records, utilization review and peer review.

In-service Education. As an institution built on the medical model, the day hospital offers an array of in-service educational opportunities for the clinical staff. These may range from self-instructional material to lectures ot full courses taken for credit or career advancement. Because the nature of adolescent work is crisis-filled, the director must be aware that such crises will always attempt to intrude upon such "luxuries" as lectures and conferences. There must be alternatives to "cancel the conference" when a crisis looms. The director must see to it that staff members are able to attend such educational meetings and that these meetings are appropriate to the task and purpose of the day hospital work. A regular clinical conference, featuring case review or outside speakers, is a hallmark of a good in-service program.

Activities Therapy. A creative and comprehensive activities therapy program is a necessity. It is preferable that these activities be therapeutic but largely *nonverbal*, since patients will also be engaged in a busy psychotherapy program. It is desirable, of course, that the activities be oriented to the distinct needs of adolescents who are living in the community rather than in the hospital. In most day hospital programs, therefore, an emphasis is placed on developing sublimations in the direction of hobbies, skills, community-oriented interests, and use of community resources.

The activities program may stress therapeutic recreation and competitive athletics as well as outings and overnight trips. It may offer a therapeutic camping excursion, ski trip, or short summer stay at the beach. Our own program has offered a "Sky Challenge for Teens Program" on a grant from the Federal Aviation Administration. "Sky Challenge" has offered flying lessons and ground school courses to selected day hospital patients (Novello, 1976).

A "survival training" program designed to teach patients basic coping skills in city life (how to use the subways, order in a restaurant, change tires, etc.) can also be a useful element. In addition, some of the more customary "hospital" activities such as art therapy, music therapy, dance therapy, psychodrama, living theater, and image groups may be offered. It is important, however, that these groups offer something different, particularly to the post-hospital teenagers, in order to avoid the realistic complaint that "it's just like it was when I was in the hospital." A skillful and creative activities therapy department enjoys distinct advantages in working with *day* hospital patients in that, almost by definition, they are less impulsive and have more ego resources available to them than inpatients. Thus, there are wider programming opportunities. Incidentally, the activities therapy department probably has a greater contribution to make in the day hospital than in the impatient program.

Behavior Modification Program. Most day hospital programs for adolescents have found it desirable to include a behavior modification component. This feature provides for a basic "behavioral management umbrella" under which the talking, psychodynamic psychotherapy can, it is hoped, flourish. Token economies, "point systems," levels of privileges and responsibilities may all be elements of such a behavioral system. The system must, of course, be adaptive to specific clinical needs of individual patients and be an integral part of the overall treatment program as prescribed by the attending psychiatrist.

In general, it is much more difficult to build an effective behavior modification program in a day hospital than in a 24-hour hospital, since the staff has far less control over the patients' activities. Again, this aspect of the program calls for staff expertise and a sensitivity to the distinct nature of the day hospital concept. Cooperation and collaboration with parents are necessary to a degree far beyond that required of parents of hospitalized adolescents.

Therapeutic Community. The day hospital movement, in general, has stressed a basic reliance on the therapeutic community concept. Many adolescent programs operate on this principle. Usually there are daily or weekly "community meetings" run by the adolescent patients but supervised by the staff. While the therapeutic community has advantages in fostering group cohesion and the maintenance of a "pro-therapy" atmosphere, it poses certain practical and philosophical difficulties for the day hospital. The adolescent patients, after all, live their lives in the larger community where successful techniques of daily coping may run counter to the philosophy of therapeutic community. While *adult* day hospital patients may be able to call upon experience and more mature judgment in making the daily back-and-forth adjustment from life "on the outside" to therapeutic community life, adolescents may find the experience frustrating and confusing. It should also be pointed out that, from a practical standpoint, the day hospital's therapeutic community (as opposed to the 24-hour hospital community) is like a sieve; there is no way, especially in working with drug-abusing adolescents, to keep a whole host of noxious, non-therapeutic contaminants out of the therapeutic community. Still, the concept has considerable merit in adolescent programs if staff is aware of the inherent limitations and if they are skillful and diligent in maintaining the virtues and expectations of the therapeutic community.

Crisis Intervention. The staff, with direction provided by the psychiatrist-director or attending psychiatrist, must be prepared to provide clinical intervention in a number of crisis situations. Classroom intervention, at the request of the teacher, is the most frequent request. In some programs, nursing staff may actually monitor classrooms on a regular basis. In others, they remain available to the teachers.

The ability to respond to crises during evenings or weekends is a crucial function of the day hospital, particularly if it truly aims to serve severely disturbed adolescents and to keep them out of the hospital. The availability of the psychiatrist and perhaps various other members of the staff can be pivotal, especially in the first month post-hospital for the youngster who has been hospitalized. Some day hospital programs require a home visit by the social worker or nursing staff prior to admission, not only for purposes of information-gathering but also to make their presence and future availability known in a very concrete and demonstrable way.

Liaison. The day hospital must maintain more active liaison with referral and disposition sources than the 24-hour adolescent hospital program. In many cases the teenagers will be in concurrent outpatient therapy with a referring psychiatrist while they are in the day hospital program. Desirable exchange of relevant information and the avoidance of "splitting" require active liaison efforts.

The adolescents may also be participating in a wide variety of other community activities while they are in the program. While it is neither desirable nor necessary that all of these activities (driver's education, karate lessons, piano lessons, part-time jobs, etc.) should be under active observation by the staff, in certain selected cases such activities may actually be *prescribed* for the patient. In these cases, the activity becomes part of the actual treatment plan and the social worker or nursing staff, with permission of the teenager and his parents, may actually visit the outside instructor or employer.

Liaison with probation officers and the court can also demand much time and attention from the staff. If the adolescent is court-involved, it is likely that he will be under regular scrutiny by the juvenile system. The hospitalized youngster is usually "turned over" to the hospital for treatment and the probation officer relies on occasional written progress reports. With an adolescent in the day hospital, however, the probation officer and the treatment team often find themselves as active partners, with frequent phone calls and meetings being necessary in difficult cases.

When the youngster leaves the program to return to a local school, the staff can provide a valuable liaison service to the public school counselor and classroom teachers. A "reentry" meeting with these individuals, held before the adolescent is discharged, can ease this transition. Some day hospital programs provide for a terminal "half-day" program where the youngster attends therapeutic activities for part of the day and journeys to his new school for classes during the remainder of the day. Liaison efforts by the staff, in these cases, are crucial to the success of the transition. Evening or after-school day hospital programs should, of course, also maintain some form of liaison with the local school.

Redl (1976) refers to the "helicopter service" function of the day hospital. This refers to the availability of the clinical program staff to the local school for crisis intervention or consultation after the adolescent has left the day hospital.

Hospital Backup. No day hospital program that seeks to treat severely disturbed adolescents can operate successfully without solid and reliable backup from a 24-hour hospital. By the nature of their problems (suicidal tendency, marginally compensated psychosis, psychosomatic problems, and a myriad of acting-out symptoms), a certain number of these youngsters will require periods of brief hospitalization during the course of their day hospital treatment. Rather than becoming discouraged, day hospital staffs generally recognize this as a fact of life and pride themselves on working with the teenager and his family toward expedient discharge and reentry into the day program. This can be accomplished, however, only if the day hospital staff and the inpatient staff work closely and harmoniously together. Although various models may be used, the most satisfactory approach is for the day hospital staff to continue working with the patient while he is in the hospital. He may continue to attend the day hospital groups and certain other activities as a device to keep him oriented to the outside community, rather than turning inward to the hospital program. Such cooperation between staffs can be jeopardized by a host of factors. Day hospital staffs usually understand the inpatient program much better than the inpatient staffs understand the day hospital, since the former have usually been recruited as experienced hospital staff members, while the latter only rarely have had day hospital experience. Day hospital staffs, therefore, know they cannot afford to cultivate a separatist attitude; they are usually quite aware of their reliance on the inpatient unit and are prepared to spend time educating their inpatient colleagues regarding the philosophy of their own program.

Disposition Planning. Because of their unique role in a "world between" the hospital and the outside community, the day hospital staff members are in a position to have a grasp of community resources that will be valuable in effecting disposition planning when the patient is ready for discharge. Considerable attention is given to this task by staff. Whereas placement from a 24-hour hospital is apt to be "temporary" (i.e., to a day hospital, another hospital, or a long-term residential treatment program), placements from the day hospital itself tend to be more "definitive," since this treatment modality is specifically for adolescents with better psychological functioning than their inpatient counterparts. This opens up many creative possibilities for suitable disposition, such as private schools, boarding schools, community schools, jobs, living at home, living in group homes, etc. Although most youngsters will require at least once weekly outpatient therapy after leaving the program, they will still be going to a much less intensely therapeutic environment. Clinical decisions for discharge readiness, therefore, must be very carefully pondered if regression and re-hospitaliation are to be avoided.

The School Component

The second major element of the overall day hospital program is the therapeutic school. Adolescents in a typical "full day" (8:00 a.m. to 5:00 p.m.) program will spend approximately four hours in the classroom. It is desirable, of course, that the adolescent student-patients be able to earn credit for completed work, especially if they will remain in the program for something more than very short-term treatment.

It is crucial that the clinical staff and the teachers maintain close liaison. Most school programs are located in the same building that houses the partial hospitalization program, which obviously enhances programming and communication.

The role of the teachers in such a program is a very important philosophical issue. Are the school and its teachers to be completely isolated and divorced from therapy? "Teachers teach and therapists therapize and the twain do not meet," might be the motto for adherents of such a model. On the other hand, there are enthusiasts of a more egalitarian model where "everyone is a therapist" and where teachers might also serve as co-therapists in group therapy and be expected not only to confront but to *interpret* patients' behaviors in the classroom.

While aware of the arguments, pro and con, for each of these models, I favor a middle course, i.e., teachers and staff work closely together and share information but distinct roles are maintained. I feel that adolescents need some important extra-parental adults in their lives to be "real people" with whom they can experiment in new emerging behaviors. Thus, teachers do not interpret or "therapize" and therapists do not teach or attempt to intervene at all in the classroom unless invited specifically by the teacher.

The fundamental organization of the school component itself has important implications. Some programs, particularly evening or weekend programs, may operate on a tutorial basis. Full-day programs, on the other hand, require much more comprehensive facilities and staffing. In these cases, the school may be organized as a branch of the local school system or the hospital may create its own private, accredited therapeutic school. The latter arrangement has obvious advantages in the areas of programming, recruitment, cohesion, and accountability. In addition, it gives the day hospital patients a certain identity as "students" who attend a private school. Thus, they can tell their inquisitive neighborhood friends that they attend "the Jones School" rather than "The Psychiatric Day Hospital"—an important face-saving device for many youngsters. (Program staff, however, should not encourage this too far; if carried to extreme it encourages a handy resistance for the adolescent patients and some parents as well: the well-known "I'm-just-here-for-school-syndrome.")

The Psychotherapy Component

Direct psychotherapy services are generally rendered by the attending psychiatrist himself, perhaps in combination with staff psychologists, nurse therapists, or social workers under his direction.

As previously noted, most day hospital programs are traditionally built around a group therapy concept. Thus, the most intensive programs might offer daily group therapy in combination with individual and family therapy.

The availability of individual therapy is important for those teenagers, mostly late adolescents, who are most capable of self-observation and of maintaining a therapeautic alliance. One immense advantage of day programs over inpatient programs is that continuity of treatment with referring outside therapists is much more of a possibility. Patients can be given time off from the program to attend such appointments. It this is undertaken, however, there must be concise prior agreement between the outside therapist and the program psychiatrist regarding their roles and the nature of their collaboration. It is usually preferable for the program psychiatrist to maintain overall medical responsibility since he sees the patient much more frequently and in a wider variety of settings; it is usually also important for him to maintains the administrative perogatives, particularly regarding behavioral expectations within the program. Other arrangements, though more complex, are workable if the outside therapist is cooperative and available to the program psychiatrist and staff.

Family Therapy. The nature of family therapy in the day hospital may differ from that in inpatient programs in several strategic ways. First of all, the parents, when all is considered, are really the day hospital's "night staff." They must be collaborators in the treatment in a way that is not required of parents of inpatients. At the same time, they are engaged as parents in family therapy by the same staff. Obviously, a "balancing act" requiring great tact and skill on the part of the clinicians is the order of the day.

Another important difference is in the amount of responsibility and participation that is expected of the parents or parent surrogates. Inpatient programs, by their very nature, take on numerous "parenting" roles. Parents may participate in family therapy but, on a day-to-day basis, it is the hospital staff that protects, nurtures, stimulates, teaches, treats, and sets limits. Day hospital staffs, conversely, generally operate on the philosophy that the "behavioral reins" must be placed firmly back in the parents' hands. Therefore, if a patient commits a serious breach of conduct, the day hospital therapist may call mom or dad at the office and ask how *they* want to handle it! The day hospital may also place increased emphasis on teaching parenting skills to the parents of its young patients, perhaps in didactic, "for parents only" groups.

In a great many cases, the single most important criterion of treatment success is the parents' willingness and ability to actively support the program's policies and goals. While parental resistance in all of its many forms is well-known in adolescent hospital work, parental cooperation is much more of a "make or break" phenomenon in the day hospital.

Although some day programs admit youngsters who are not living with their parents (and some programs even operate in conjunction with their own group home), inevitably they require some form of ongoing participation on the part of a designated parental surrogate. Attempting to treat seriously disturbed adolescents without closing this loop is usually doomed to failure.

Like the group and individual therapy, the family therapy is generally set within a psychodynamic mode although "systems" and "communication" approaches are becoming more and more prominent. Whatever the philosophical underpinnings, the family therapy may be offered on an individual basis (especially for crisis-ridden, "needy" families) or on a multiple family group basis (which is a powerful treatment modality particularly suited to programs featuring a therapeutic community concept).

PATIENT SELECTION

If the day hospital is truly to be utilized as an alternative to in-patient hospitalization, criteria of admission should be *inclusive* rather than exclusive. When an adolescent patient is brought to the hospital, the admitting psychiatrist should first ask, "Can he be admitted to the day hospital?", rather than, "Which inpatient unit do we send him to?"

Day hospital programs develop their own specific admissions criteria based on the program's task and purpose, as well as its overall capabilities. Generally, these criteria fall under six headings:

1) *Sufficient Impulse Control.* The adolescent patient must have sufficient ego capabilities and impulse control to travel back and

forth from home each day and to maintain himself safely in the community and in the program. This criterion, therefore, would rule out actively suicidal, destructive, and homicidal youngsters. Psychotic adolescents may also be ruled out, but only if they are not in sufficient control. Adolescents with uncontrollable "acting-out" difficulties, such as a runaway tendency, are also better treated, at least initially, in the more secure inpatient environment. Similarly, teenagers with substance abuse problems that seriously hinder their daily functioning cannot be treated in the day hospital. It should be pointed out, however, that the amount of impulse control required for the day hospital is a matter of degree and often rests on the experienced judgment of the admitting psychiatrist. If the program is to really succeed as an alternative to the hospital, the psychiatrist must, first and foremost, be intimately aware of the capabilities of the day hospital and willing to take some calculated chances. One related subcriterion that may help him in this judgment is the adolescent's ability to utilize helpers, in a verbal mode, to assist in his own efforts at impulse control.

2) *Intercurrent Medical Illness.* Any intercurrent medical illness, whether or not it is directly related to the primary psychiatric diagnosis, must be manageable on an outpatient basis. If the day hospital provides on-site medical consultation, as it should, some fairly serious medical problems can be managed without inpatient referral. Adolescents suffering frequent asthmatic attacks or bouts of colitis, for example, have been managed successfully. Anorexia nervosa can also be treated in the day hospital in a great many cases.

3) *Parental Support.* As noted previously, the program must have a commitment of support for its policies and goals from the patient's parents or parental surrogates. Their active participation in program maintenance and in the family therapy is a matter which is so crucial that, without such a commitment, it is doubtful that the treatment can succeed.

4) *Appropriate for School.* Since the therapeutic school is an integral part of the full day program, the patient must be suitable for the school. When this is in doubt, an evaluation by a diagnostic/prescriptive teacher prior to admission is indicated.

5) *Transportation.* Day hospital intake staff, unlike their inpa-

tient counterparts, must know about the area's public transportation system. Careful consideration must be given to such logistical items. How will the patient get there in the morning? What time will he have to leave home? Is he capable of transferring on subways or buses? How will he return home? Will it be dark when he gets home? If so, is there any danger? Is travel time so excessive that it interferes with homework, part-time jobs, or family activities? These and a host of other related questions must be addressed. Some programs furnish their own transportation; while this may make some of the previous questions less germane, it may add other roles for the program administrator—transportation director and unofficial mechanic.

6) *Finances.* Financial considerations may, unfortunately, play a large part in determining a youngster's suitability for the program. Always a factor in private psychiatric treatment, the financial consideration is often made more difficult by insurance companies which paradoxically prejudice coverage in favor of the more costly full-hospital program. Therefore, some decisions must regrettably be made not on clinical grounds but on financial factors. It is not unusual, for example, for a patient's insurance plan to provide for 100% of inpatient costs (which may be on the order of $150 per day or more) and nothing at all for day hospital (which may be on the order of $50 per day). Even if 75% or 80% coverage for the day hospital is provided, many families simply cannot afford the 20% or 25% "out of pocket" costs. The adolescent, in these cases, may be hospitalized at a greater monetary cost to his insurance company—and at a greater psychological cost to himself and his family.

There are two additional criteria that have little to do with the patient himself but which should always be addressed in this type of work with adolescents. First, how will a particular teenager "fit" with the other youngsters in the program? The cultural fit may be much more important than the clinical fit. For example, a "straight" teenager may be scapegoated by a group of "streetwise" adolescents; a black youngster may be scapegoated by white teenagers or vice versa; an early adolescent may be ostracized by a group of middle or late adolescents; a teenager with physical deformity may be too threatening to other youngsters' narcissism, etc. The other criterion is one of staff morale. The day hospital work itself can be draining.

How much energy does the staff have at the moment for a particular patient?

The reader will note that, thus far, this discussion of patient selection has *not* stressed the importance of specific diagnostic entities in determining day hospital suitability. This is done with design. Most highly structured programs find that DSM II or DSM III diagnoses are simply not very useful in determining admission suitability. Basically, the day hospital can handle virtually any type of patient that the 24-hour hospital would normally treat (schizophrenia, major affective disorders, borderline syndromes, severe neuroses, depression, psychophysiologic disorders including anorexia nervosa, character disorders, substance abuse problems, etc.) if the abovementioned criteria are met. In some cases the day hospital will clearly be taking a chance, especially on the "judgment" criterion of impulse control. The day hospital *should* take chances. With adequate hospital back-up, teenagers who fail in the day program can be quickly hospitalized.

The day hospital that boasts a "success rate" of 90% or higher, in all likelihood, is playing it too safe. It may be handpicking its patients and denying admission to a number of youngsters who, then, must be hospitalized. Particularly for a program whose mandate is to act as a front-line alternative to 24-hour hospitalization or to shorten hospital stays of seriously disturbed adolescents, a "success rate" of 75%-80% is a worthy goal.

One final word about patient selection. It is often believed that adolescent day hospital patients are "easier" to treat than inpatients. This is a myth. If anything, they are more difficult. The staff attempts to treat basically the same type of adolescent who is seen in hospitals without the important advantages of the hospital, such as locked units, seclusion rooms, parenteral medication, environmental control, 24-hour staffing in shifts, etc. For the adolescent, the ultimate bulwark between the day hospital and 24-hour hospitalization is the skill and devotion of the day hospital personnel themselves.

STAFFING

In an attempt to explain the always high attrition of clinical staff on adolescent inpatient units, Meeks (1977) said that "many are called but few are chosen." If, indeed, the inpatient staff is a chosen breed, the day hospital staff must not only be "chosen" but "anointed."

The day hospital is not the place to learn about adolescent psychiatry—unless one is a student. A day program that attempts to treat seriously disturbed adolescents can only be successful if it is staffed by the most experienced and skilled staff. Therefore, most day hospital directors recruit only from among staff members who already have worked at least two or three years in an adolescent inpatient unit. The other vital criterion is the staff member's ability to exercise sound clinical judgment and to use himself or herself as a therapeutic agent. While this is always important in staff selection, it is imperative in the day hospital.

For example, an inpatient nurse can turn a disturbed patient over to the next shift at the end of eight hours and go home secure in her knowledge that the patient is safe. The day hospital nurse, on the other hand, may have to make very difficult decisions everyday at 5 p.m., i.e., should this youngster go home at all today? Was his casual reference to death really a communication of suicidal intent? Should his parents be alerted? Are they home tonight? Should the attending psychiatrist be consulted? In this case the nurse may decide to meet privately with the youngster and then send him home; she may also lose some sleep that night.

One additional criterion for staff selection may be the person's ability to relate to individuals and agencies outside of the hospital, since special liaison, disposition planning, and referral development skills are usually required in day hospital work.

The question of staff professional qualifications, numbers and organization is complex. After-school and weekend programs, almost by definition, serve the less disturbed adolescent and, therefore, may have less of a medical model orientation. These programs are often largely staffed by psychiatric social workers and psychologists with part-time psychiatric supervision. The full day programs tend heavily toward the medical model and may, in fact, be basically organized as a nursing unit, with a psychiatrist director, a nurse unit administrator, other nurse-clinicians, and psychiatric technicians. In these programs, social workers and psychologists may also be involved in clinical roles, often with the families. I have found that the full day program optimally requires, in addition to the director and nurse administrator, one nurse-clinician (or social worker) and one psychiatric technician for every eight to ten patients. Attending psychiatrists may relate to the program in a number of ways.

The number of activities therapists may vary widely depending on the degree of "specialization" in the hospital's activities therapy department. Secretarial and administrative support must also be sufficient for a smooth-running program. The staffing pattern for teachers, of course, is the responsibility of the school program.

In closing this section, it must also be noted that day hospital staffs usually have an "image" problem with their inpatient colleagues. They have usually been specifically recruited for their positions. Because they are the most experienced people in the hospital, they are likely to be the highest paid for their positions. They do not work nights or weekends (except in crises) and may have some "free time" during the teenagers' usual vacations or breaks. They are imagined to be working with the "easiest" patients. These factors can lead to jealousies and resentments from their inpatient colleagues. Some day hospital staffs react by isolating themselves from the rest of the hospital, while others may develop a kind of elitist attitude. Both stances, of course, are counterproductive. One of the best ways of maintaining close working relationships is for both staffs to work together in some ways; this provides better continuity of patient care and promotes mutual respect for each other's roles.

OUTCOME STUDIES

While a number of excellent outcome studies have been conducted in adult day hospitals, there are no comparable studies specifically in the field of adolescent programs. This is unfortunate and should be corrected. In reviewing the adult studies the reader should be cautioned that, while some overall conclusions relative to adolescent programs are suggested, the results cannot be uniformly applied to adolescents.

In one of the first outcome studies in the day hospital movement, Kris (1961) found that when patients otherwise destined to be admitted to a psychiatric hospital were randomly assigned to a day hospital instead, they fared as well as or better than the inpatients.

Zwerling and Wilder (1964) demonstrated further that the day hospital could be an alternative for a large number of actively disturbed patients. They reported a study showing that two-thirds of a group of newly admitted inpatients who were randomly assigned to a day hospital were actually accepted for treatment at the day hospital. The remaining third were rejected and were treated in the inpatient setting. Of the patients accepted by the day hospital, 60% never required complete hospitalization. In other words, approximately 35% of patients who otherwise would have entered the hospital were completely treated in the day hospital. These earlier studies in adult psychiatry demonstrated that the day hospital *could* be an alternative; the question of whether it *should* be an alternative has more recently been addressed by other investigators.

Herz, Endicott, Spitzer, and Mesnikoff (1971) not only found that over 20% of hospitalized patients could be treated in the day hospital but that, on virtually every measure used to evaluate outcome, there was clear superiority of day treatment over inpatient treatment, i.e., day patients had shorter stays, fewer readmissions, etc. These investigators speculated as to why the day hospital results were superior and concluded that the day program apparently avoids the "regressive" features associated with total hospitalization and that the day patients have a greater opportunity to maintain healthy areas of functioning. The Herz et al. study was unique in that there was no special program for the day patients, i.e., they were treated in some physical location by the same staff and participated in all ward activities along with the inpatients. The authors pointed out that the crucial variable, therefore, was the basic distinction that the day patients were only on the ward 8:30 a.m. to 5 p.m. on weekdays. The authors further speculated that a special day hospital program would even further enhance the superiority of the day hospital results. In answer to the question of whether the day hospital *should* be utilized, the authors answered that "optimal treatment requires a well-integrated inpatient, day, and outpatient program. Close monitoring of the status of an acutely disturbed patient should be routine and should allow for early transfer to day hospital status . . . too often, patients are left to languish in a hospital until a lengthy evaluation period is completed. After a patient has been admitted to an inpatient service, *if there are no con-*

traindications to day hospitalization, day care is preferable to continued inpatient care."

In a carefully controlled study, Washburn, Vannicelli, Longabaugh and Scheff (1976) extended these outcome findings by assessing a greater span of variables, by following patients over a longer period of time and by extending the earlier findings to a middle- and upper-class population. Washburn's study was designed to study the relative efficiency of inpatient versus day hospital treatment for a population of patients, all of whom began their treatment with inpatient hospitalization and who, under usual hospital procedures, would have continued in that setting. In addition, he studied a group of "usual" day hospital patients for comparison with the randomized day hospital group.

Washburn et al.'s study strikingly demonstrated that day treatment is preferable to inpatient treatment in four distinct ways: 1) Subjective distress—day patients enjoyed quicker symptom resolution and sense of well-being. 2) Community functioning—the randomized day patients improved more than the inpatient controls not only during the first six months of the study but during the second six months as well. 3) Subjective burden to family—families of day patients were more satisfied with the treatment location and they felt less "burden." This confirmed the findings of Hoenig and Hamilton (1966) that extramural management creates a greater degree of family tolerance. The day center family was able to avoid the shame, guilt, anxiety, and even stigma that, unfortunately, is still associated with complete hospitalization. Washburn also felt that since the family is constantly making adjustments to the presence of the "patient," it avoids the sudden readjustments that occur in the inpatient's family each time he returns home. Finally, it could be pointed out that day patients, by sustaining some role in the family, continued to be of some value within the family system. 4) Costs—total direct charges to the day patients were significantly lower than for the inpatients due, of course, to the lower cost of staffing an eight-hour program rather than a 24-hour inpatient unit.

As stressed at the beginning of this section, these studies have been carried out largely with adult patient populations. Treating adolescents in a day setting is a somewhat different matter. Adolescents are almost always more problematic due to developmental factors that limit their ability to form a therapeutic alliance and that favor "acting-out" as symptom expression and defense. The family's active collaboration and participation are even more crucial in working with adolescents and the complexity of extraneous relationships with peers, teachers, probation officers, etc., make the task more difficult.

Until a controlled study, such as Washburn's, is applied to the adolescent day hospital, we will not have definitive answers. Nevertheless, some speculations can be offered. On the basis of three years' experience in both a "free-standing" and a "hospital-based" full day program, I believe that an outcome study comparing the adolescent day hospital and adolescent inpatient hospital would show results similar to those from adult outcome studies in many important respects. The differences are probably of degree rather than kind. For example, while adult studies suggest that 20-35% of inpatients could have been directly admitted to the day hospital, this figure is undoubtedly somewhat lower with adolescents. I estimate that 10-20% would be more accurate.

Adolescent length of stay, on the other hand, would be longer than for adults, just as adolescent in-hospital stays are usually longer because of developmental and other issues. Also, the length of stay would, of course, vary widely with the nature and purpose of the program itself.

Washburn et al.'s findings are fairly consistent with the experience of professionals in the adolescent day hospital. The youngsters do seem to feel less subjective distress and more acceptance of the treatment modality; also, community functioning does appear to be enhanced. Families, while they are more satisfied with the treatment location, may, in fact, feel *more* burden than families of inpatients, at least in the early phase of treatment. Finally, there is no doubt as to the cost-effectiveness of the day hospital over the 24-hour hospital. Even in cases where an adolescent might be treated over a longer period of time in the day hospital, the total financial saving can be considerable since daily costs are generally only 25-40% of those of inpatient treatment. Thus, at the cost of one "hospital month" an adolescent may be treated intensively for three or four months in the day hospital.

In summary, there is rather compelling evidence from studies in adult psychiatry that the day hospital can offer both superior clinical outcome and superior cost-effectiveness over inpatient treatment for a large spectrum of patients judged considerably sicker than patients who are usually considered for that setting. Although comparable studies do not yet exist in adolescent psychiatry, I feel that many similar advantages exist for the adolescent day hospital over adolescent inpatient treatment. Yet, if this is so, why is the day hospital the most underutilized resource in all of adolescent psychiatry?

UNDERUTILIZATION

It has been pointed out repeatedly that the underutilization of partial hospitalization programs represents one of the great paradoxes in our current health care delivery system (Wilder, 1971; Fink, Longabaugh and Stout, 1978). Given the special developmental advantages where adolescents are concerned, as well as the clinical effectiveness and fiscal advantages of day hospital programs, it seems paramount to explore the causes of this underutilization. Such an exploration is all the more imperative at a time when medical costs are coming under increasing societal pressure and when court-mandated requirements for psychiatric treatment of adolescents in the "least restrictive environment" make it increasingly difficult to hospitalize youngsters involuntarily.

The question of underutilization can be explored from several perspectives.

The Adolescent Patients

The underutilization is surely not the fault of the adolescent patients themselves. Insofar as they can or will accept *any* form of psychiatric treatment, adolescents overwhelmingly prefer the day hospital to inpatient treatment. In fact, this is one of the strongest inherent advantages of adolescent day hospitals.

The Parents

In discussing adult programs, several investigators have stressed that families enjoy greater "treatment satisfaction" in the day hospital as opposed to 24-hour programs (Wilder, Levin and Zwerling,

1966; Herz et al., 1971; Herz, Endicott and Spitzer, 1977). Washburn et al. (1976) have particularly found that, for the partial hospitalization families, the patient's illness imposed less burden during the initial hospital-based treatment and that, with time, this "subjective cost" further decreased, whereas it actually *increased* during the comparable following period for inpatient families.

I have found that, while there is general parental preference for the adolescent day hospital, there are some unique parental resistancs. First of all, many of these youngsters are embroiled in developmental conflicts with their parents. By the time the matter is brought to psychiatric attention, a terrible toll in family functioning may have already been taken. Many parents, in these cases, do, in fact, wish to have their youngsters hospitalized. If they are given a day treatment option, they will find rationalizations, such as transportation problems, to favor a hospitalization. In some cases, of course, parents simply feel overwhelmed and drained; they may express a preference for the 24-hour program and, in such cases, it may actually be the preferred initial treatment modality. In other cases, parents, while harboring conscious or unconscious preferences for hospitalization, may *not* express a direct preference to hospitalize their youngster. (They may be burdened by guilt; they may be intimidated by their hostile youngster, etc.) If given a day hospital option, they may accept it and then manage to sabotage the treatment efforts (mostly on an unconscious basis) by various forms of non-compliance with the treatment plan. Of course, when the adolescent must then be hospitalized, it is made to look as though it was the adolescent himself who failed, in spite of his parents' willingness to give him "one last chance to make it outside of the hospital."

Parental "burden" in the adolescent day hospital has not been systematically studied. I believe that the burden is greater than the family burden reported by Washburn et al. in their study of adult patients because of the nature of the adolescents and their often parent-directed conflicts and because of the need for intensive parental involvement in the treatment. Yet, this "burden" is only onerous at certain points in the overall treatment course and, in general, parents do prefer the day setting over the inpatient setting.

Surely, parental burden or parental resistance, even when it does exist, is not a strong enough factor to explain the gross underutilization of adolescent day hospital programs.

The Staff

Day hospital staffs are invariably enthusiastic and almost evangelical about their work. Most of them zealously accept the challenge of keeping adolescents out of hospitals. Experienced nurses and psychiatric technicians identify with the day hospital "movement" and are conversant with its growing scientific literature. Part of this stems probably from the fact that they are underdogs (i.e., the day program is underutilized) and they have a mission to develop the full potential of their programs. However, day hospital staffs, usually with good reason, may see themselves as "stepchildren" to the inpatient programs, which may be better funded by the hospital administration. This can stimulate cohesion and purpose but, if it continues, may result in disillusionment. Although staff turnover is much lower in adolescent day hospitals than in inpatient units, good people do sometimes decide to leave when they sense a lack of commitment from the hospital administration. Yet, in summary, the staff itself is undoubtedly the day hospital's strongest asset.

Poor Patient Selection

Day hospital psychiatrists and their staffs are increasingly aware that, although they may have admissions criteria firmly in their own minds, they are sometimes remiss in communicating them to referring psychiatrists. This omission contributes somewhat to the underutilization problem. Too often, referring psychiatrists and agencies are simply unaware of the capabilities of the day hospital. Severely disturbed adolescents (psychotic, depressed, acting-out, etc.) are referred directly to inpatient units without consideration at all of the less restrictive day program. This problem can be alleviated if the day hospital not only has established admissions criteria but can communicate these clinical and logistical criteria adequately to their referral sources. Studies to determine the "profile" of the successful adolescent day hospital patient should be conducted and the findings should be properly communicated.

The Concept

Is the concept of an adolescent day hospital itself simply unworkable? There are some professionals who would answer "yes" to this question. Adolescent day hospitals have been attempted and abandoned in a number of cases because the work was just too difficult. It is not uncommon for psychiatric hospitals to start an adolescent day hospital only to become quickly discouraged at the prospects of attempting to treat seriously disturbed youngsters outside of a hospital.

The work, as noted throughout this chapter, is indeed difficult but I firmly believe that the basic concept itself is sound. In some cases the problem is the implementation of the concept. Sometimes the founders are unclear as to the purpose and task of their fledgling programs in the first place; they fail to develop a cogent philosophy. In other cases, a philosophy exists but the program staffing and overall design are incompatible with the overall goals of treatment. Nevertheless, these failed attempts should not be too harshly criticized. After all, there are very few models for successful programs in the United States. Would-be developers are too often left to "rediscover the wheel."

Insurance Carriers

There is no question that medical insurance companies contribute to the underutilization of the day hospital. Typical coverage for psychiatric illness is prejudiced in favor of the more costly inpatient treatment. The federal government's high option plan, for example, provides 100% coverage for inpatient but only 80% for the day hospital. Imagine the paradox when the treating psychiatrist approaches a hospitalized adolescent and his parents and says, "You've worked hard in the hospital and there's a way that we can shorten your hospital stay. How would you like to be discharged, live at home, and just come in every day for treatment?" Before the appreciative patient and his parents can answer, the doctor continues, "There's good news and bad news. The good news is that the day hospital costs are much lower than the hospital charges. The bad news is that it will cost *you* more money!"

A good many insurance plans provide virtually no coverage for day hospital treatment but may provide 100% coverage for a short (30-day) psychiatric hospitalization. In these cases the patient and his doctor may truly be standing precariously between Scylla and Charybdis. In the first place, adolescents who require full hospitalization generally require more than 30 days. But the coverage does not apply to day hospital care. If the amount of dollars of coverage in such a hypothetical case could be applied to the day hospital, the same teenager could be treated intensively for three or four months.

I have had the experience of recommending the day hospital for an adolescent in such a situation, i.e., the insurance plan provided 100% coverage for inpatient services, but nothing for day treatment. When the president of the insurance company was reached by phone and told that not only could we keep one of his subscribers out of the hospital but that we could also save his company at least $100.00 per day over several months if he would permit day hospital coverage, the president was not impressed. He answered that, unfortunately, there was no provision in the contract and there was nothing he could do. Furthermore, he was not going to encourage day hospital coverage in the future because there was a "danger" in funding any new programs at all, even if it appeared that they might save money. As he saw it, and as the insurance industry generally views it, such coverage would stimulate growth and utilization of the day hospitals without any guarantees that there would be a simultaneous reduction in the utilization of inpatient facilities. The end result, in their way of thinking, would be overall increased, not decreased, costs and higher premiums to their subscribers.

Advocates of the day hospital must be aware of these arguments and prepared to answer them with compelling financial as well as clinical answers. Cost-effectiveness studies already completed may, of course, be cited but additional community-based studies would be helpful.

In the short run, one can accomplish more in convincing the subscribing groups rather than their designated carrier that they should include specific day hospital coverage in their overall plan. In the long run, insurance companies might be urged toward psychiatric coverage equal to general medical benefits with, perhaps, a fixed annual dollar amount, with the patient and physician free to select the most clinically appropriate setting and treatment modality.

But are the insurance companies really the single most important factor in the underutilization of the day hospital? Longabaugh et al. (1974) studied the question and concluded that undercoverage was certainly a factor, but, even when insurance coverage *is* available, the day hospital is underutilized.

Hospital Administrators

Hospital administrators usually think in terms of "bed occupancy." There are numerous historical and practical reasons for them to do so. As long as external pressures (insurance companies, lending bankers, accreditation agencies, etc.) and internal pressures (the board of directors, for example) force them in the direction of filling hospital beds, they have little incentive in promoting *alternatives* to their inpatient units. Some forward-thinking administrators have grappled with this problem and have found ways to provide comprehensive inpatient and day hospital programs which are both clinically and fiscally sound. While they are to be commended, hospital administrators, in general, continue to be a factor in the underutilization of the day hospital.

The Psychiatric Profession

Investigators who have studied the underutilization of day hospitals (Herz et al., 1971; Finzen, 1974; Washburn et al., 1976; Fink et al., 1978) invariably point to the psychiatric profession itself as the most important variable. Psychiatrists, by virtue of their training, understandably think of the hospital first when they are faced with treating a seriously disturbed patient. After all, since there are relatively few day hospital programs in the United States, very few psychiatrists have had any experience with that treatment modality. Very few residency programs, for example, offer rotations in a partial hospitalization program.

Where adolescents are concerned, the problem is compounded. Adolescents can be difficult to treat. Few psychiatrists in a busy private practice setting are able to respond to the many crises of severely disturbed adolescents and their families. Hospitalizing these youngsters or sending them off to therapeutically-oriented boarding schools or residential programs is often a handy expedient.

Some investigators have found that physician uneasiness with the day hospital, even when one is available as an alternative, is also an important factor. These clinicians may feel that the day hospital does not offer intensive therapy or that there is too great a risk. On the other hand, psychiatrists who have had direct experience in day hospitals tend to utilize them to a greater degree than those who have not had the experience. For example, in the study of Fink, Longabaugh and Stout (1978), 10 psychiatrists screened patients for possible entry to a day hospital program; of the 10 physicians, three were experienced in day hospital work while the other seven had no experience. The three with experience admitted 86% of the patients during the study! This observation is consistent with the contention that the nonclinical biases of clinicians are as important in determining treatment site as the patient's psychopathology (Washburn et al., 1976).

Inpatient psychiatrists may be slow or reluctant to transfer hospitalized adolescents to the day hospital unless certain administrative or organizational factors encourage them to use the day hospital. There are some subtle reasons to explain this phenomenon. After all, hospitalized adolescents, together with their families, are certainly among the most difficult treatment challenges in psychiatry. Such youngsters on admission are apt to be angry, hostile, and defiant. Their families exhibit a wide array of resistances. Yet, after the "resistance phase" of treatment and when they have achieved better impulse control and have established the beginnings of a therapeutic alliance with their doctor, these adolescents are a professional pleasure to treat.

The psychiatrist, quite understandably, may not be terribly anxious to transfer this delightful patient to the day hospital so he can admit to his inpatient unit the next angry, hostile, defiant teenager on the waiting list!

Overriding all of these factors, fortunately, is the psychiatric profession's ultimate concern for the welfare of its patients. All of the intra-professional reasons for their underutilization can be overcome. If psychiatric residency programs offered more training opportunities in day hospital, more psychiatrists would clearly utilize them in their later professional work. If the experience of their patients is successful, psychiatrists will bring pressure to bear on hospital administrators and third party agencies to stimulate utilization.

FUTURE OF THE ADOLESCENT DAY HOSPITAL

I am cautiously optimistic about the future of the adolescent day hospital. A number of developments appear to be coming together in such a way as to encourage the day hospital movement. Hospital and medical cost containment is an urgent professional and social issue. The day hospital has proven its cost-effectiveness over 24-hour hospitaliation. Where adolescents are concerned, there are mounting judicial mandates to treat youngsters in the "least restrictive environment." The day hospital as the most intensive level of psychiatric treatment other than the hospital itself will be the logical alternative for a number of adolescents when the "least restrictive" criterion is scrupulously applied.

The psychiatric profession continues to scrutinize itself and its treatment effectiveness with increased emphasis on peer review and clinical accountability. The day hospital has been proven superior in clinical results to the 24-hour hospital in several studies and it seems inevitable that the profession will act favorably upon that information.

Believers in the adolescent day hospital concept, however, cannot simply sit back and wait for these events to happen. They can make things happen by working hard in several distinct areas:

1) encouraging day hospital experience in psychiatric residency training;

2) educating psychiatrists and other referral sources to the capabilities of the day hospital;

3) educating the public;

4) lobbying for fiscal support from insurance carriers (and their subscribers) and for inclusion of appropriate partial hospitalization benefits in any National Health Insurance program;

5) undertaking research specifically in the field of *adolescent* day hospital in order to scientifically demonstrate its value.

REFERENCES

FINK, E. B. LONGABAUGH, R., & STOUT, R. The paradoxical underutilization of partial hospitalization. *Amer. J. Psychiatry*, 135:713-716, 1978.

FINZEN, A. Psychiatry in the general hospital and the day hospital. *Psychiat. Quart.*, 48:489-495, 1974.

HERZ, M., ENDICOTT, J., & SPITZER, R. Brief hospitalization: A two-year follow-up. *Amer. J. Psychiatry*, 134(5):502-507, 1977.

HERZ, M., ENDICOTT, J., SPITZER, R., & MESNIKOFF, P. Day versus inpatient hospitalization: A controlled study. *American Journal of Psychiatry*, 127:1371-1381, 1971.

HOENIG, J. & HAMILTON, W. The schizophrenic patient in the community and his effect on the household. *Amer. J. Psychoanal.*, 26:165-176, 1966.

KRIS, E. Prevention of rehospitalization through relapse control in a day hospital. In M. Greenblatt (Ed.), *Mental Patients in Transition*. Springfield, Illinois: Charles C Thomas, 1961.

LONGABAUGH, R., McAULEY, T., IMERMAN, L., & WESTLAKE, R. The acute day hospital as an alternative and/or addition to inpatient psychiatric treatment. Butler Hospital Treatment Evaluation Series (No. 6), Providence, R. I., 1974.

MEEKS, J. Personal communication, 1977.

NOVELLO, J. R. Sky challenge for Teens. Use of Flight Training as Adjunctive Therapy in Adolescent Psychiatry. Report to Federal Aviation Administration, Education Branch, 1976.

REDL, F. Personal communication, 1976.

WASHBURN, S., VANNICELLI, M., LONGABAUGH, R., & SCHEFF, B. A controlled comparison of psychiatric day treatment and inpatient hospitalization. *J. Consult. Clin. Psychol.*, 44(4):665-675, 1976.

WILDER, J. F. Discussion of Herz, M. I., Endicott, J., Spitzer, R. L., et al.—Day versus inpatient hospitalization: A controlled study. *Amer. J. Psychiat.*, 127:1381-1382, 1971.

WILDER, J. F., LEVIN, G., & ZWERLING, I. A two-year follow-up evaluation of acute psychotic patients treated in a day hospital. *Amer. J. Psychiat.*, 122:1095-1101, 1966.

ZWERLING, I. & WILDER, J. F. An evaluation of the applicability of the day hospital in treatment of acutely disturbed patients. *Israel Annals of Psychiatry and Related Discipline*, 2:162-185, 1964.

14

Hospital and Residential Treatment of Adolescents

WILLIAM M. LORDI, M.D.

Slavson, approximately twenty years ago, made the interesting observation that in the approach to adolescent therapy, one cannot use strictly a psychoanalytical model, but rather one has to use a para-psychoanalytical model. This implies that adolescence is a time of life where the individual is "becoming" and therefore there is some growing capacity for introspection and some capacity to distance one's self from problems. The process is by no means complete. An alternative, not within the awareness of the adolescent, also has to be supplied to the youth to make his or her choice; therefore, more active intervention of the therapist is needed than in the more classical analytic treatment situation.

DEVELOPMENTAL CONSIDERATIONS

Adolescence is a time when the individual is passing through innocence, lack of awareness, lack of insight, lack of capacity for in-depth introspection, toward a rehearsal for adulthood. Youths need continuous support, guidance and direction in the formation of these skills. Lichtenstein, in a new book, *The Dilemma of Human Identity*, states that in the prestructural state of development human beings have to create themselves in accordance with an image passed on to them primarily by the imprinting by their mothers. We define adolescence as a time when all these earlier forces become manifest. It is important in evaluating and recommending treatment that we are acutely aware of the youth's actual state of development. There are many examples of personality arrest, failure to form love object relationships, absence of role modeling supplied the youth and many other important developmental errors. These, of course, can also be exaggerated by substrate problems such as biological deficits, via a variety of physical illnesses and diseases that have occurred during early development and extend to the time of evaluation. Examples of these are epilepsy, diabetes, organic brain syndrome and other general physical disturbances.

HOSPITAL TREATMENT

This chapter will emphasize hospital treatment. Some comments on residential treatment will also be offered in an attempt to make differentiations between *hospital* treatment and *residential* treatment and to define the kind of youth who benefits from these two distinct types of programs.

The hospital is the most intensive treatment center, where there are gathered a host of treatment disciplines using the medical model. There are the psychiatrists with their medical background, neurological background and training in psychiatry and child psychiatry. There are the child psychologists who, in addition to their training in general psychology, have training in child psychology, evaluation and treatment of youth. There are the psychiatric social workers who specialize in the area of family and children and the impact that the larger social network has on the child and family. There are the pediatric psychiatric nurses who, in addition to their nursing skills, are aware of the special developmental tasks in health and illness, both physical and emotional. The pediatrician's expertise is with the physical well-being of his patients. The mental health technicians are aware by training and experience of the special developmental tasks of adolescents and how these are affected by familial, psychological and emotional problems. The psychoeducational staff are concerned with putting together the specific educational and learning program to meet the needs of the child, interdigitating it with total program so that the teenager can keep pace with the work of adolescence—learning in school. These specially prepared teachers have a knowledge not only of the developmental tasks of adolescence, but also of the effects that emotional, physiological, familial, organic and learning disability factors have on the youth. There are recreational therapists and occupational therapists who, because of their special training, provide a treatment program as part of the total therapy and work with the adolescents basically at a nonverbal level providing outlets for alternate expressions of problems and feelings, as well as for alternate solutions. The overall strategy and pace are managed by the adolescent psychiatrist.

It is of paramount importance that adolescents be carefully selected for hospitalization. There is a lingering aura that hospitals are places where one goes to die—psychologically as well as physiologically. Hospitalization is also a mark that the family system can not maintain, sustain, or repair the adolescent's problem. One has to deal with the concomitant, sometimes subtle, sometimes blatant, undercutting of hospital treatment on the part of the family system, since this family system may be defective, is possibly involved in the production of the problems in living that the youth presents, and may need the adolescent to live out the family pathology.

The model of the Joint Commission on Accreditation of Hospitals evaluation system is a very useful one. It points out that one should utilize the minimum amount of penetration into the alteration of the life-style of the adolescent as well as the therapies that are needed to restore him to good functional capacity in a reasonably well functioning family unit. This implies, therefore, if the identified problem can be handled on an outpatient basis, this should be done. Therefore, we might consider a hierarchy of intensity and level of restriction: outpatient treatment, day hospital, acute hospitalization, long-term hospitalization, forensic care and residenial treatment. One recommends one of these "levels of treatment," based on a consideration of the nature of the problem, its meaning for the individual in the system in which he is involved and the community in which he lives and its resources. The psychiatrist should attempt to select the least disruptive and restrictive therapy but also one that has the best chance of restoring the youth and his family to the community in a functional fashion so that the community resources can be mobilized as soon as possible to meet his needs on an outpatient basis. This kind of clinical decision-making is, of course, difficult. The adolescent psychiatrist must draw upon his own experiences and skills, his knowledge of potential treatment resources and, above all, his careful evaluation of the individual adolescent patient.

The problem of proper "level of treatment" recommendations is social, emotional, and socioeconomical. It also impacts on the philosophy of medical practice, the community and third party payers. It is important that we maintain credibility with ourselves, with our colleagues, with our patients, with our community-at-large, with the third party payer systems, and with peer review systems. It is obvious, therefore, that we are simultaneously relating to many segments of the total community. The day is gone when we simply treat the patient for his intrapsychic disequilibrium. A systems approach is necessary for the psychiatrist to thoroughly understand the task at hand and what must be done to adequately meet the needs, first, of his young patient and, after, of the many other "interested parties."

Criteria for Hospitalization

As indicated, hospitalization represents the result of careful screening of the necessary level of intervention to meet the problem as it presents itself, recognizing that adolescence is itself a time of a great many crises with wide mood swings, problems with differentiation and individuation from the family, flight back into childhood, rebellion, distancing and many other acute and intense phenomena. Sometimes, seemingly in the blink of an eye, an adolescent has an acute psychotic decompensation and an outpatient facility cannot contain him because of the danger to himself or others or his panic is so great that he could exhaust very quickly the physical, as well as the emotional, strength and endurance of any family.

The American Psychoanalytic Association, The American Academy of Child Psychiatry, and the American Psychiatric Association have attempted in their manuals for peer review to establish those criteria that are the minimum necessary for appropriate hospitalization. This represents the distillate of experience from at least these three vantage points, bringing together in-depth experience from the disciplines represented and also providing a basis for documentation which subsequently validates the necessity for admission and retention of the patient in the hospital. Periodic utilization reviews help determine the length of hospitalization if it goes beyond the usual and customary. At the same time, criteria must satisfy the demands of the family, third party payers and other agencies and users of hospital services.

It is interesting to note that the State Department of Mental Health and Retardation in Virginia has also set forh new regulations covering the rights of youth. It requires all hospitals to set forth their areas of competence, the goals of their facility, the diagnostic evaluations available, the procedures for referring patients, the procedures in emergency referrals, and the conditions under which hospitals will accept referrals from other resources. One must also state their limitations. It specifies that all patients must be admitted by a member of the medical staff and must have an admitting diagnosis to justify admission. It also recognizes that there are special care patients where one diagnosis may not be so clear initially but at least establishes the necessity for protecting these young patients from themselves and from society in general until a more exact diagnosis can be arrived at.

It is obvious from this that the government, as well as the professionals and third party payers, is very interested in the proper hospitalization of patients so as to protect the well-being not only of the individual but of society-at-large and to best use the resources that are available.

Many of us in adolescent psychiatry are acutely aware of the various health service boards in local communities and on the state level which are attempting to bring some order out of the previous chaos where there seemed to be an open marketplace burgeoning with all kinds of services. Now there is accountability not only in terms of the number of beds but also in the kinds of beds and kinds of services to maximize community use of its facilities and to take a regional, statewide and nationwide approach to this third largest of all industries—the health industry.

Another dimension which has developed out of our necessity to justify hospitalization and diagnosis is that we are beginning to see patterns where some emotional disturbances recur partially because of our lack of understanding of treatment goals and patterns. For example, we have noticed in our own setting that many of our admissions have been in three or four acute, intensive treatment units;

in reviewing records of these adolescents we found that their remissions were good and the reasons for discharge were good. When one studies their longitudinal pattern, however, it becomes apparent that another level of hospitalization was indicated after the acute phase was satisfactorily completed. Many of these adolescents really required an *intermediate,* rather than *acute,* length of treatment.

It is important to note that, diagnostic category for diagnostic category, we have noticed, in the practice of adolescent psychiatry, that the length of stay and the duration of symptoms are about three times that of the adult. In order to understand these phenomena we must again utilize a developmental perspective. Adolescence is a time of intense becoming, of going extremely rapidly from one developmental task to another with an ever-increasing number of developmental complexities: the forces for emancipation, the impact of hormonal drives, new social tasks, new body, no experience, a society that urges prematurity on the young, adult accomplishments and ideas, and a general shortening of the developmental stages in adolescence over the necessity to reestablish the youth in his developmental track according to his ability and opportunities in the community, the family and the entire system.

The Intermediate-Length Hospital Program

We have developed the intermediate-length hospital care of nine to 24 months for those youths who have demonstrated by their life pattern and by their use of therapy on many levels that there is a recurrence of maladjustment. The intermediate-length program makes greater use of the adolescent as his own agent of change; this is emotionally and cognitively dwelt on in therapy and in innumerable daily interactions with the staff as well as within the peer patient group itself.

While human beings cannot be measured with the exactitude of sheets of timber, nevertheless we are beginning to arrive at operational and functional criteria for admissions and continued hospitalization. The human rights issue has entered the picture in a very interesting way over the past several years, indicating that adolescents have their own rights which must be jealously guarded and must be considered even in view of the degree of personal disturbance that they may be undergoing at the time. This dimension has not often been considered in the past. Hospitalization has very often seemed to be at the pleasure of the family, the community, and sometimes the hospital, if not the doctor.

We are also beginning to evolve a more satisfactory understanding of the natural history and development of problems in living of youth. This kind of compelling, self-imposed responsibility also helps us understand that the human condition is predictable, to some extent modifiable, and treatable to a greater degree than we ever imagined in the past. This does not in any sense rob the professions of the arts they practice, nor does it cast human beings in concrete. However, this kind of thoughtful approach not only validates diagnosis and length of stay, but also compels us to delineate careful therapeutic plans which expedite the process of self-knowledge, treatment and alteration of old adaptive patterns in order to effect new attitudes that contain understanding of the self, healing old wounds, the formation of new alliances in families, and ultimately the resolution of the presenting symptoms. The outcome, it is hoped, will be better mental health than was previously enjoyed, even before the crisis came to the surface.

It must be noted that the acute hospital itself encourages regression in the service of growth. The intermediate-length hospital poses a different philosophy, one which says in effect that the teen-aged patient has demonstrated the capacity to effect important changes in his life, and that the treatment team holds him to that responsibility. It is true that in this program the youths have to spend a good deal of time dwelling on what has happened to their unmet needs out of childhood or even in previous therapy. They eventually come to accept the challenges of taking responsibility, identifying their problems, working out plans to meet these problems with their psychotherapist, setting goals, and setting time-frames in which to accomplish them. They are helped to get in touch with sources of their own strength and power and to master their identified problems as they work on them in individual and group psychotherapy, in the therapeutic community meetings and in all their therapeutic activities, whether they be psychoeducational, or activity therapy.

Case Report

John Smith, a boy of 15, began to experience increasing anger, depression, and school failure. He was staying out late at night and was involved in alcohol and substance abuse. This seemed to have emerged starting early in his thirteenth year. Simultaneously, his father had been away in the service. The mother had several young children to look after. With nothing coming in emotionally, the mother began to drink and see other men. When this came to light, the husband and wife had a good fight over it. They both made promises. This began to impact on the child, who was going through his own separation-individuation and the anxiety of adolescence. He was introduced to pot smoking. He began to skip school. As if to retaliate, the father began to have his own affair when he was stationed back home. This was not lost on John. There began to be more rounds of anger. The problem came to a head when the boy was involved in an accident where he was driving a stolen car under the influence of alcohol. This was an almost naked suicide attempt on his part. In addition, he apparently had been using unidentified drugs. He was admittedly out of control. When seen for psychiatric interview, he presented himself as being psychotic with many paranoid features and much regression. We later learned that what he had used was LSD.

Because of the nature of the problem and the danger to himself, he was admitted on an emergency basis. Because of his paranoid ideation, his degree of violence, and the fact that he was a small boy but taking a banty rooster approach to the world, he was placed on a closed unit. After his admission, which involved a careful history-taking from the parents, it emerged that there was essentially no medical underpinning—that is, no brain or biological problem. John was a boy who had achieved in school until he was 13 and was of above average intelligence. There was no apparent learning disability. The blood and urine tests gave us some lead on the nature of the drug problem. The acuteness of the decompensation and the background led us to believe that we were not dealing with a schizophrenic break but rather with an acute drug-induced psychosis.

He was placed on Thorazine in a closed unit. He had a physical examination as soon as he settled down. He was examined by the psychologist. A social case history was done. Daily rounds were made by the psychiatrist, who also managed his medication and made modifications of the day-to-day program.

The boy became visibly nonpsychotic in about a week. The elements of depression became more apparent. He made several suicide gestures. He cut himself. He displaced a great deal of his anger and hostility onto the staff, feeling that we had no business interfering with his life, especially with his desire to kill himself. The family was seen in ongoing couples therapy. The child was seen in intensive therapy. The balance of the medical workup, which included an EEG, neurological, SMA-14, chest x-ray, psychoeducational evaluation, was within normal limits.

A staff conference was held at the end of the first week and the diagnosis was reviewed; the diagnosis was "depressive reaction with an acute drug-induced psychosis in an adolescent of bright intellectual endowment with serious familial dysfunction." We felt the child's assets were his brightness, his early vague attempts to find some solution to his problems in living, and the fact that the family was galvanized into action. We felt that the problems, in addition to a highly dysfunctional family, were his depression, his inability to find better methods of coping with his anger and despair, his sense of abandonment, his sense of neglect, his great anger turned on himself and his low self-opinion. John's size was an important problem to him.

The treatment plan, in addition to getting the patient out of the acute psychotic episode with medication, was to continue the individual psychotherapy and introduce group psychotherapy. John was put on a point system to earn his way out of the closed unit. We were concerned about how he cared for himself, how he demonstrated caring for others and how he was willing to participate in the general life of the therapeutic community. We set goals of his being able to help the other youths on his unit during the many therapeutic "raps" that took place, in addition to his participation in group and individual psychotherapy and his willingness to start conjoint family therapy. There was a great outpouring of hostile feelings by the youth when he was with his parents. They returned some of the anger toward him but began to share with him their sense of guilt and sense of sadness over their participation in his problems and their inability to meet their own problems in living.

After an initial period of medication for three weeks, the medication was discontinued. He did need some medication for sleep on several occasions. In all, John was hospitalized for six months. During that time there was some evidence of physical growth, which delighted him. He began to see his mother and father as real human beings. He learned of their backgrounds and the deprivation they had growing up, and why they could stand separation so poorly. He could often parent them. They saw him as a remarkable boy, being able to sense things "beyond his years." John was able to work his way out of the closed unit in a period of one month. His psychological tests showed that he was definitely college material. The educational tests showed that he had not paid attention, had been truant but was not far behind academically. In six months he was functioning at grade level.

The treatment, predictably, was difficult. John went through periods of rage. He was able to recognize how he displaced onto people and how he especially picked on men and how protective he was of women. Ultimately, he was able to face his anger at his mother for what she had done and how she had betrayed the father. He was able to share his anger about the poor role model his father provided, as well as his father's absence. While there were many steps forward, there were some steps backward. John tried to hide behind "coupling" with a girl in the program which so often happens with youths in a hospital. He was able to be faced with the fact that "coupling" itself represents a "hide-behind" (i.e., defense) which made it unnecessary for him to face the work of his problems in living. He reluctantly gave up his love affair and the relationship developed into that of friendship. John was also able to deal with another boy coupling with this ex-girlfriend.

Throughout this program three meetings were held where all staff members involved—the teacher, the individual therapist, the group therapist, the attending psychiatrist, the mental health team, members of the unit team—met and discussed in-depth with John and his family the identified problems, the steps that were being taken to deal with the problems, the progress that was being made, and the long-term planning. There were daily psychiatric rounds and supervision of the therapist by the consulting psychiatrist on a weekly basis. There were weekly meetings to discuss the progress on the unit, conducted by the team under the leadership of the psychiatrist.

During his stay John was reviewed twice by an independent child psychiatrist who judged that he was not ready to leave the hospital at the time of the two reviews. A month before he left, plans were made for him to return to school. Inasmuch as he lived in another community, he was referred to a psychotherapist in his own community. Complete records were made available and the progress he had made academically was shared with the school system. He was asked to come back a month after he left. A conjoint session was held at that time. On discharge it was felt that the prognosis was good.

The Therapeutic Community

The actual treatment of the adolescent in the hospital is a multi-faceted, interdigitating program. The basis is the therapeutic community. As a youth comes out of a system where he was in no small part shaped and molded and helped to become maladjusted and disturbed, so, too, he must come into a system that is highly organized and therapeutically oriented.

Therapeutic community is a baseline. By this it is implied that the actual organization and functioning of the unit on which the youngster lives, the hospital in which he is treated and the various facets of the program must all be carefully mixed. When a child is admitted, depending upon the degree of disturbance, he is placed on the locked unit or open unit, and he is put into a system of behavioral "levels" whereby he has an opportunity to concretely measure his own progress. Specific treatment and behavioral goals are immediately established. The patient is part of a "community."

In our setting, the units are organized as follows: locked unit, children's unit, and three adolescent open units. There are daily therapeutic community meetings which are led by team leaders and therapists. The locked unit has two meetings a day. The orientation of these meetings is existential. They deal with the everyday details of living—what is going on in the unit, what is going on with the individual, the problems he or she is having in the immediate environment, what the group is doing about it and how they are reacting to the individual. All of this happens in the context of a problem-oriented record wherein the assets of the individual are determined from the outset, problems are delineated, and the ultimate goals are set and plans to achieve these goals are set forth. These are reviewed with the individual adolescents after the first week, and periodically thereafter. The goals are changed according to the changes that occur in the patient, i.e., the recognition of further problems and the dropping out of old problems.

The Psychotherapy

In addition to the therapeutic community, the individual is seen in individual therapy on the average of four times a week by his individual psychotherapist. There is a contract between the individual therapist and the youth taking place wherein an alliance is formed to work on and through the problems. There is also group psychotherapy, which takes up the role of the individual as a member of a group, a family and a system. Most, but not all, adolescent patients are able to utilize group therapy. All of these treatments are under the direct supervision of the attending and consulting psychiatrist, who also has the responsibility for managing medications and prescribing all of the psychotherapy.

There is also ongoing therapy with the parents and, as soon as it is feasible, the teenager joins in the conjoint family therapy to reestablish the psychological homeostasis in the family or to work toward his separation and integration into yet another family, if, indeed, this is indicated.

Education Program

The first step is a thorough psychoeducational evaluation to determine grade level, as well as specific strengths and deficits. The educational program itself is remedial for those who have learning disabilities but progressive for those adolescents who can benefit from a more intensively "academic" program. We attempt to realistically plan the psychoeducational program so that those who can benefit from a terminal high school program are put in that track; those who are best prepared for a general educational diploma and vocational rehabilitation are placed in that track; and those that can go to college are in yet another track. The program is also prepared to deal with emotionally disturbed, learning disabled, and brain damaged adolescents as well as those with a variety of dyslexic and central processing problems.

Activities Therapy and Psychiatric Nursing

To implement and complement all of these programs there are also the nontalking therapies which utilize a variety of activities, games, and nonverbal expressive interactions to promote the working on and the working through of feelings. In a hospital setting, the role of the pediatric nurse is extremely important. She not only oversees the medication and the physical well-being of the children, but assists the pediatrician in following each of the children medically from routine physicals to immunizations, infections, injury and other medical problems that the child brings in with him or that arise in the course of his stay. The psychiatric nurse has the key role in providing leadership to the mental health technicians on the unit as they undertake the important moment-to-moment management of the youth in the program. The mental health technicians by and large are young college graduates and college students whose ultimate goal in their own lives is usually to head toward one of the helping professions. Not only do they contribute their considerable intelligence and their vitality, their process of growth and their role modeling, but they are also a major interface source to the youth. They are the part of the treatment team that does many of the one-to-one "raps," and oversees all the activities under the supervision of the nursing service, which, in turn, are guided by the consulting psychiatrist.

It is always important in intermediate-length hospitalization as well as intensive care hospitalization to have a good Career Development Program that prepares those adolescents who by reason of age, education and ability are best suited for the world of work. This very often obviates the necessity of returning to nonproductive school and a resurgence of problems. This is where Career Development has its finest hour.

The Medical Record

The ebb and flow of activity and the complexity of the interaction is recorded in daily psychiatric notes, daily nursing notes and mental health technician notes, weekly psychotherapy notes, educational notes, activity therapy notes, and the psychoeducational notes. The overall document is the medical record. Eventually this is the biography of the child as he moves through the treatment process.

The Family

In addition to the above, every attempt is made to involve the family, if humanly possible, on a once-a-week basis. Most of the families are seen once or twice a week. It is true that about 10% of the families do all they can to abandon their children to the hospital. Many of the families have been hurt, bruised and disap-

pointed and have felt misled and used. Many of them have illnesses
and pressing problems in their own right. Separation itself permits
families to gain some distance from the patient, allowing them to
begin to work on their own problems in living and their interaction with their children which eventuated in the variety of mal-
adaptations and problems. Many heretofore unrecognized forces
come to light. Family therapy is the usual and customary form of
psychotherapy that we aim for with the adolescent after he is involved in his own therapy and the family has become sufficiently
involved to understand the goals of treatment. Most of the families
are willing to participate. It is difficult and often painful, but
exhilarating, as they see both their teenager and themselves change
and grow.

Success Rate

It is hard to estimate the success rate. It is important to note that
many adolescents need an intensive hospitalization experience followed by an intermediate-length hospitalization. A good deal of the
failure of hospitalization at times is that it does not take into account that one can help in important remission, healing and real
personality structural change in a short-term, six-to-nine-month
program. But for many adolescents it is simply insufficient. A large
number of teenagers need to go on to a different form of hospitalization, the intermediate-length form of hospitalization, where the
process of structural change can be continued. Such an intermediate
program places more of the responsibility for change on the individual. Discharging the adolescent to home to be followed on an
outpatient basis is often not sufficient. This abrupt change in "level
of treatment" is contraindicated for many severely disturbed adolescents. The evidence for this is that most of the adolescents in the
intermediate-length treatment program have previously been in
three or four other intense hospitalizations. Their remissions have
not been lasting. They obviously require something more than an
acute length of hospital stay.

Treatment Termination

An adolescent is ready to leave the hospital when he is capable of
socializing with his peers on a reasonably successful level consistent

with his age. He is ready to leave when there has been amelioration of the symptoms; when he has identified his problems, and has begun to work profitably on them and is able to sustain himself during some crises; when he is feeling hopeful about the ultimate prognosis and when he is returning to a family that also feels hopeful and willing to continue work. There are few, if any, adolescents who could go from a hospital to home without some level of outpatient treatment. Some adolescents may require transfer from an acute-length hospital program to an intermediate-length program.

In the intermediate-length hospitalization, the goals are structural change so that the chances for recurrence of the long-standing emotional problems which made it impossible for the teenager to adjust on an outpatient basis, or to maintain himself even after acute hospitalization, are greatly diminished. For termination from such a program, therefore, the psychiatrist essentially looks for a higher level of personality function. In addition, there should be a viable family relationship or a viable substitute family relationship established. Also, the presenting symptoms should have remitted, and the adolescent should be achieving consistent with his ability and prepared for the world of work or college if he is a late adolescent.

RESIDENTIAL TREATMENT

A residential program offers treatment for an extended period but at a less intense and less "psychiatric" level of care. Resocialization and psychoeducation are common goals in such programs. The adolescent is helped to find a variety of new adaptive techniques that enable him to cope with the community when he returns. These adolescents usually are psychiatrically very much less disturbed and belong in neither the intense psychiatric treatment hospital nor the intermediate-length treatment hospital.

Intermediate-length hospitalization, on the other hand, is for those adolescents who have had important psychiatric structural problems and where perhaps there has been some amelioration due to their having been in an acute and intensive treatment setting. This by no means enables them to attend a regular school or return to their own community. They can best benefit in the long run from continued intermediate psychiatric treatment which features ongoing supervision by experienced adolescent psychiatrists, psychiatric nursing personnel, activities therapists, and specially trained educators. The program is based upon the concept of therapeutic community but also contains elements of behavior modification, as well as the full spectrum of psychiatric hospital services including medication and pediatric consultants. The program meets hospital standards and submits to both internal and external review.

Residential programs, while they might provide some level of psychiatrist involvement, are not hospitals. They are more therapeutic than boarding schools but less intense and less medical than hospitals. They are an appropriate "level of care" for some adolescents.

SUMMARY

The advantages of hospital treatment lie in the intensity of focusing on the psychiatric needs of the adolescent. The intermediate-length hospitalization treatment is of obvious benefit in that it obviates the necessity for repeat acute hospitalization or substituting repeat acute hospitalization for the needed, longer-term hospitalization. It is suited for adolescents who may have resolved more superficial "presenting problems" (such as overdose or runaway) in an acute phase of treatment but who are plagued with serious underlying personality deficits. They, therefore, require continued intensive treatment on an intermediate-length basis with goals that stretch far beyond mere symptom resolution, i.e., structural change, better social adjustment and school performance, vocational preparation and the realignment of family relationships. There are few disadvantages to hospitalization if one keeps in mind the basic issues: 1) adequate penetration level for the problem at hand, 2) the developmental stage of the adolescent, and 3) the psychological status of the family.

The indications for hospitalization are 1) when the adolescent cannot function adequately socially, 2) when the community resources cannot be mobilized to help him, 3) when there is an acute crisis endangering the adolescent or the family system, and 4) when other less restrictive forms of therapy have been tried and have not met the needs of the adolescent.

Intermediate-length hospitalization is required when the degree of structural pathology in the child will not lend itself to quick remission with medication and short-term intensive psychiatric treatment.

Residential treatment is indicated where socialization, education and discovering alternative adaptive patterns are the treatment of choice.

REFERENCES

AMERICAN MEDICAL ASSOCIATION. *Peer Review Manual I and II*, 1972.
AMERICAN PSYCHIATRIC ASSOCIATION. *Manual of Psychiatric Peer Review*, September, 1976.
COMMONWEALTH OF VIRGINIA. *Rules and Regulations for the Licensure of Private Psychiatric Hospitals*. Department of Mental Health and Mental Retardation, 1978.
JOINT COMMISSION ON ACCREDITATION OF HOSPITALS. *Accreditation Manual for Psychiatric Facilities Serving Children and Adolescents*. Chicago, 1974.
LICHTENSTEIN, H. *The Dilemma of Human Identity*. New York: Aronson, 1978.
MEEKS, J. *The Fragile Alliance*. Baltimore: Williams and Wilkins, 1971.
SLAVSON, S. *Group Psychotherapy for Children*. New York: International Universities Press, 1968.
WHITAKER, J. K. & TRIESCHMAN, A. E. *Children Away From Home*. Chicago: Aldine, 1972.

Index